Alternative Treatments
for Fibromyalgia and
Chronic Fatigue Syndrome

We dedicate this book to Dr. Paul Brown, without whose loving care neither of us would have been able to pull off this book. We also dedicate this book to our compatriots in pain, especially those who shared their stories with us.

Ordering

Trade bookstores in the U.S. and Canada please contact:
Publishers Group West
1700 Fourth Street, Berkeley CA 94710
Phone: (800) 788-3123   Fax: (510) 528-3444

Hunter House books are available at bulk discounts for textbook course adoptions; to qualifying community, healthcare, and government organizations; and for special promotions and fundraising. For details please contact:

Special Sales Department
Hunter House Inc., PO Box 2914, Alameda CA 94501-0914
Tel. (510) 865-5282   Fax (510) 865-4295
e-mail: ordering@hunterhouse.com

Individuals can order our books from most bookstores or by calling toll-free
1-800-266-5592

Alternative
Treatments
for Fibromyalgia
& Chronic Fatigue Syndrome

*Insights from Practitioners
and Patients*

Mari Skelly and Andrea Helm

Hunter
House
PUBLISHERS

Hunter House Inc., Publishers
P.O. Box 2914
Alameda CA 94501-0914

Library of Congress Cataloging-in-Publication Data

Skelly, Mari
Alternative treatments for fibromyalgia and chronic fatigue syndrome : insights from
practitioners and patients / Mari Skelly and Andrea Helm.
p. cm.
Includes bibliographical references and index.
ISBN 0-89793-272-2 (cloth) – ISBN 0-89793-271-4 (paper)
1. Fibromyalgia—Alternative treatment. 2. Chronic fatigue syndrome—Alternative
treatment. I. Helm, Andrea. II.Title
RC927.3 .S54 1999
616.7'4—dc21   99-036226

Project credits

Cover Design: Peri Poloni   Book Production: Hunter House
Editor: Laura Harger   Production Director: Virginia Fontana
Indexer: Kathy Talley-Jones   Proofreader: Lee Rappold
Publicity Director: Marisa Spatafore   Special Sales Manager: Sarah Kulin
Acquisitions Editor: Jeanne Brondino   Publisher's Assistant: Georgia Moseley
Customer Service Manager: Christina Sverdrup
Order fulfillment: A & A Quality Shipping Services
Publisher: Kiran S. Rana

Printed and bound by Publishers Press, Salt Lake City, Utah

Manufactured in the United States of America
9 8 7 6 5 4 3 2   First Edition   00 01 02 03

Contents

Acknowledgments ix

Foreword by Dr. Paul Brown xi

Introduction ▪ Our Story 1

The Questionnaire 7

Chapter 1 ▪ The Diagnosis 9

Formal Diagnosis and Treatment of Fibromyalgia:

    Dr. Philip Mease 17

A Patient's Story: Ann A. 20

Fibromyalgia and Myofascial Pain Syndrome:

    Dr. Devin Starlanyl 22

A Patient's Story: Tom O. 27

Formal Diagnosis and Treatment of Chronic Fatigue Syndrome:

    Dr. Dedra Buchwald 30

A Patient's Story: Karin L. 34

Chapter 2 ▪ Symptoms of Fibromyalgia and
Chronic Fatigue Syndrome 37

A Patient's Story: Lucy J. 42

Chapter 3 ▪ Conventional Therapies 45

Chapter 4 ▪ Osteopathy and Chiropractic Therapies 52

Chiropractic Technique: Dr. Robert Freitas 55

Getting Relief with Osteopathy: Dr. Cathy Lindsay 59

A Patient's Story: Barbara M. 61

Chapter 5 ▪ **Chinese Medicine** **65**

Acupuncture: Sara Wicklein 68

A Patient's Story: Ellen J. 71

Tai Chi and *Chi Kung*: Kim Ivy 74

Chapter 6 ▪ **Mental Health and Spirituality** **77**

Psychotherapy and Chronic Illness:

　　Maureen Sweeny Romain 90

A Patient's Story: Jill M. 93

Spiritual Counseling and Chronic Illness:

　　Cornelia Duryeé Moore 97

A Patient's Story: Diane K. 103

Chapter 7 ▪ **Work and Vocational Therapy** **106**

Vocational Rehabilitation: Don Uslan 115

Chapter 8 ▪ **Natural Healing and Nutrition** **119**

Eating for Optimum Health: Joleen Kelleher 125

A Patient's Story: Erin P. 130

Naturopathy: Dr. Rebecca Wynsome 133

A Patient's Story: David A. 136

Chapter 9 ▪ **Exercise and Physical Therapy** **139**

Movement Therapy: Eduardo Barrera 144

A Patient's Story: Sherry J. 149

Physical Therapy: Dr. Kim Bennett 150

A Patient's Story: Betty M. 155

Yoga: Vijay Elarth 159

A Patient's Story: Rebecca H. 162

Chapter 10 ■ Other Healing Options 165

Craniosacral Therapy: Cherste Nilde 170

A Patient's Story: Becky R. 173

Massage Therapy: Noreen Flack 176

Chapter 11 ■ The Narcotics Controversy 180

Medical Treatment with Opiates: Dr. Michael Young 183

A Patient's Story: Melinda N. 187

Medical Marijuana: Green Cross 190

A Patient's Story: Annie D. 196

Chapter 12 ■ The Future of Fibromyalgia and
　　　　　　　Chronic Fatigue Syndrome 200

Self-Management Techniques: Dr. Kate Lorig 203

Psychological Aspects of Chronic Pain: Dr. Dennis Turk 205

Sleep Dysfunction and Fibromyalgia: Dr. Carol Landis 209

New Directions in Chronic Fatigue Syndrome Research:
　　　Rich Carson 212

Chapter 13 ■ Legal Considerations 217

Protecting Your Legal Rights: Morris Rosenberg 224

A Patient's Story: Hilary S. 228

Resources 237

Glossary 242

Drug Trade Names 253

Bibliography 255

Notes on Contributors 258

Index 263

Acknowledgements

Thanks to Ann Adam and Gene Nelson, who were so supportive in helping us get started. To the providers who gave so freely of their time and assistance; to Elaine Dondoyano, for her tireless work in transcribing many hours of tapes; to Diane Kerner, for the flyer that sent patients our way; to Anton Moentenich, for providing the photos for the book; to the Fibromyalgia Mutiny Group, for their great support and friendship; to Ellen Jablow, for helping us with technical and computer support and for being the Goddess of the Glossary; to Val Gardner, who helped get the iMac going; to Nick Albion, for his invaluable computer expertise; to Alex Dittmar (www.spacecow.net) who set up our Web site; to David Brachtenbach, who also gave us helpful computer assistance; to Jeanne Brondino, who made a huge leap of faith and took a chance on two unknown writers; and to Jolanta Irla, a pharmacist who answered all our many questions.

We also acknowledge a local publisher, who was kind enough to point out that our manuscript was "bleak and depressing."

Mari

Thanks to my parents, Dick and Vivian Skelly, and my brother Richard and his family, for their constant support, and especially Gayline Skelly, for her advice along the way. To my special friend Peggy Rader, who is always on my side. And to my partner, JoAnn McMillen, R.N., who provided invaluable technical expertise and always believes in me. A special thanks goes to Jill Birnberg, M.S.W., and Robyn DeSautel, D.C., who took care of me even when I had no money. Their love and commitment to their patients is awesome! I would also like to recognize Tammie Tays, who manages her own chronic illness with grace and humor. She reminds me that when the going gets tough, the tough go to garage sales.

Andrea

Thanks to Gary Joseph, who always keeps me guessing; to Laura Bowers, for eight years of friendship; to Patrick Mills, whose constant harassment kept me writing when I wanted to quit; to my family members, who never let me get too conceited; to Jessica Maxwell, who told me I had talent; to Mark Worth, who taught me that truth can bring down giants; to Janice Chapman, for her many years of friendship; to Stan Webb, Tracey Yost, and Michael Sheldon, for putting up with me as long as they did; to my treatment providers, for helping me on my road to recovery; to Dr. Sandra Jo Counts, who helped me handle my pain; to Tresa Savin, my new sister in crime; and, finally, to all the people who wouldn't call me, publish me, date me, or hire me.

Foreword

Fibromyalgia (FM) is a clinical condition characterized by widespread pain and fatigue associated with a myriad of other symptoms. Although initially believed to affect a limited number of people, FM is now reported to affect as much as 10 percent of the population in certain regions. This percentage is steadily increasing, in all likelihood because of increased reporting as a result of greater awareness by patients and physicians alike due to increased media coverage and the emergence of new Internet groups and support groups.

Chronic fatigue syndrome (CFS) is an illness characterized by severe, persistent fatigue. Some of its symptoms are similar to those of FM, and a certain percentage of people with FM also have CFS. Not all people with FM have CFS, and vice versa.

The American College of Rheumatology definition for diagnosing FM relies solely on subjective criteria. Thus, to be diagnosed with this condition, a patient only has to verify that pain occurs upon the physician's application of pressure to at least eleven designated areas on the body. However, because patients with FM and CFS do not "look sick," many physicians deny the existence of these very real conditions. Others believe these are psychiatric conditions, but this is not the case. (Although 25 percent of patients with FM are depressed, FM and depression are not synonymous.)

There are currently few tests that can confirm the presence of either FM or CFS through objective findings. For this reason, obtaining an accurate diagnosis is often difficult. In our current climate of managed care, doctors may be reluctant to order expensive testing. Additionally, patients with FM or CFS are hard-pressed to get the care they need. Unfairly, the burden has been placed on patients to prove they are ill.

Although there is no cure for these chronic conditions, many patients improve with the help of low-dose antidepressants, muscle relaxants, sleeping aids, analgesics, or a combination of medications. Drugs normally used to prevent seizures, such as clonazepam or gabapentin, also help alleviate symptoms. Since traditional medicine isn't always successful, many patients experiment with alternative therapies and natural products, with some success. Many of these alternative therapies are discussed in this book.

Aerobic conditioning (in moderation), physical therapy, biofeedback, acupuncture, chiropractic care, hypnosis, and cognitive behavioral modification techniques [see the Glossary for a full description] have also offered relief to many people. There are many other remedies, some of which haven't been studied in clinical trials. However, this doesn't mean they are not useful.

Patients with other diseases that cause chronic pain are given narcotic analgesics if they don't respond to less potent pain relievers. The same should be true for FM patients, but this is not always the case. Treatment with narcotics, when necessary, can alleviate the pain, fatigue, and cognitive problems, permitting patients to feel and function better. Methadone, a synthetic narcotic analgesic, may be particularly useful for patients who have not responded to non-narcotic medications.

The possible presence of thyroid disease, growth hormone deficiency, sleep apnea, other medical conditions, and some medications, which can all cause symptoms similar to those of FM and CFS, shouldn't be overlooked. In one study, eleven of forty-six women diagnosed with FM had another disorder that actually caused their pain.

Advances in research on and treatment of FM and CFS are progressing so rapidly that even specialists have difficulty keeping up with them. For this reason, I am very excited about this book, *Alternative Treatments for Fibromyalgia and Chronic Fatigue Syndrome: Insights from Patients and Practitioners*. I know both authors personally and recognize their courage, dedication, and integrity. They have produced a book both intimate and practical. Are you interested in learning about the role of nutrition, Chinese medicine, spirituality, or craniosacral work in treating these disorders? Want to know whether FM and CFS are actually the same condition? Are you interested in learning about how trauma can cause FM? These and many other questions are answered eloquently by a group of carefully selected experts and by people living with these disorders. This is an extremely useful book that will help all sufferers of FM and CFS to lead a better life.

Dr. Paul Brown

Paul B. Brown, M.D., Ph.D., is a renowned fibromyalgia treatment specialist and a rheumatologist in private practice in Seattle, Washington. He is a clinical associate professor at the University of Washington and lectures at conferences on the West Coast.

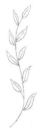

Important Note

The material in this book is intended to provide a review of information regarding fibromyalgia and chronic fatigue syndrome. Every effort has been made to provide accurate and dependable information. The contents of this book have been compiled through research and in consultation with medical professionals. However, healthcare professionals have differing opinions, and advances in medical and scientific research are made very quickly, so some of the information may be disputed or become outdated.

Therefore, the publisher, authors, editors, and professionals quoted in the book cannot be held responsible for any error, omission, or dated material. The authors and publisher assume no responsibility for any outcome of applying the information in this book in a program of self-care or under the care of a licensed practitioner. The information contained in this book should not be used as a substitute for the care of a medical doctor. If you think that you have some of the symptoms discussed in this book, check with a licensed physician. You can also call the Arthritis Foundation for a list of specialists in your area (see the Resources section in the back of this book). Always consult your physician before making any changes to your current treatment plan.

Introduction:
Our Story

FIBROMYALGIA (FM), which predominantly affects women, is a syndrome of widespread pain characterized by tender points found on at least eleven out of eighteen specific places on the body that are tender when pressed. Imagine being beaten up, having food poisoning, getting the flu, and not sleeping for a week— all at the same time. You hurt all over. Your stomach is churning. Your bowels are in knots. Your brain is foggy, and you're exhausted. This is what it's like having FM, every day, all day, maybe even for the rest of your life.

Chronic fatigue syndrome (CFS) is a specific illness characterized by severe, persistent fatigue, and it is often associated with difficulties in sleep and concentration, aching muscles and joints, headaches, sore throat, and depression. Over the last few years, the CFS community has lobbied for a name change to better describe the reality of the condition. The suggested acronym is CFIDS, which stands for "chronic fatigue and immune dysfunction syndrome." While this new acronym does describe the syndrome more accurately, for the purposes of this book, we will continue to use CFS, since that is the term with which most people are familiar.

FM and CFS are invisible disabilities. If you looked at us, you might not believe that we are suffering from an incurable, painful illness. But looks can deceive. The Pigeon River, which flows through North Carolina and Tennessee, is a wild and beautiful river. You might never guess that, below its surface, it contains enough dioxin to kill an entire community. It has been poisoned by effluents from a paper mill upstream, and signs along its banks warn residents not to swim in it, drink the water, or eat any seafood taken from it. Increased incidences of cancer can be traced along its banks. We don't look sick, either, and this is one of the many difficulties that people with FM and CFS face—looking well but feeling like hell.

Mari Skelly was first diagnosed with FM in April 1994, when she was thirty-one years old. While she had faith in her care team and followed their treatment plan, she also was interested in trying "alternative" therapies and anything else that might help alleviate her pain. She went to numerous physicians and providers, looking for ways to manage the constant pain in her feet, legs, and back. After three years, her primary-care provider finally referred her to a place that was considered to be on the cutting edge of pain management. She went in looking for pain relief, but only got a pain in the neck for her troubles.

She arrived early in the morning to fill out forms. The biggest was the Minnesota Multi-Phasic Personality Inventory, which is structured much like the SAT test, with hundreds of multiple-choice questions. She worked on this paperwork between constant visits from doctors and therapists. However, every time she was interrupted, she would become very confused and lose her place on the form, marking her responses incorrectly. Later, after receiving a copy of the session transcript, she learned that the psychiatrist had said she'd tried to skew her results to appear more functional than she actually was. (As she was trying to get into a pain clinic, Mari later wondered, why would she purposefully try to appear as though she didn't need it?) It did not occur to her at the time to let the doctors know about the difficulty she was having in trying to complete the questionnaire; since they were the "experts," wouldn't they understand the cognitive difficulties facing a person with FM?

At the end of the day, Mari met with all the doctors and therapists, who told her that she was not a "good candidate" for the pain clinic, because typically they had had little luck in helping a person who did not have "clear goals for the future." They wondered, too, if she had enough energy to go through the pain clinic's day-long, strenuous physical therapy program.

As Mari sat there, dumbfounded, a doctor told her that her insurance didn't cover the entire cost of the program. Mari stammered that she could probably come up with the extra thousands of dollars herself if necessary. The program director then told Mari point-blank to leave and find out if she had sufficient funds to cover the program's cost. Then she could get back to him.

Mari had hoped, when she arrived, that she would learn self-management skills that would help her deal with her pain. Instead, she left in tears. Was this all about money? Had her doctors believed that her HMO insurance covered the program's cost or if she had paid the cost out of her own pocket, Mari probably would have been admitted—whether the doctors believed they could help her or not.

Looking back, Mari says now that if she ever does anything like that again, she'll be sure that she understands everything up front instead of blindly trusting that a profit-driven health-care system will do what's best for her recovery.

Sadly, Mari's experience is a perfect example of the problems that FM and CFS sufferers face when trying to get help: disbelief, misinformation, and grief from the very people we seek out for treatment. And Mari's story was not the worst we heard while doing interviews for this book. She could have given up, and for a while she was very discouraged and upset, but it only made her more determined to learn about other treatment options.

At the age of thirty-four, Andrea was rear-ended in an automobile accident. Less than a year after the accident, she was diagnosed with both FM and CFS. When she could no longer work full-time, she was fired from her well-paying computer-industry job. Inability to pay rapidly rising medical bills destroyed her hard-earned credit rating. Friendships withered and died because she could no longer expend the energy necessary to keep them. Cherished hobbies—dancing, gardening, reading, writing, furniture refinishing, haunting thrift shops and flea markets—bit the dust one by one. Andrea's world narrowed to little more than medication refills, doctors' offices, massage therapy appointments, acupuncture sessions, and feelings of guilt that her boyfriend had to take care of most household finances and chores.

Luckily, her FM doctor referred her to a pain-management specialist. Thanks to the miracle of drugs such as Neurontin and Oxycontin, Andrea no longer lives in constant pain and despair. Now she's able to take a walk in the park and marvel at the beauty of a sunset, which she took for granted so many times before she became ill. She is often able to count her blessings instead of dwell on her sorrows. She is able to live "in the moment" and have faith in her body's ability to heal.

Andrea also hopes to effect change in the laws governing those disabled with chronic pain. She's learned that people with FM and CFS face many kinds of discrimination in employment and obtaining disability benefits. We should not be fired from our jobs when we honor doctors' orders to cut hours. We should not have to wait years to get Social Security disability or private insurance benefits. We should not have to hassle with HMOs, whose agenda preserves their financial bottom line. We should not have to deal with ill-informed social-service workers or fill out endless forms in triplicate. If nothing else, Andrea's illness has served as on-the-job training in learning to stand up for her rights.

■ ■ ■

After our diagnoses, we read everything we could get our hands on about our conditions. But we were always looking for a book that documented both the treatment plans of trained professionals and personal testimonies of people living with FM and CFS. We wanted a book that had it all. After not finding one on the shelves, Mari began to imagine writing one of her own. We hoped to prevent others from having to learn the hard way about the pitfalls of the health-care system, as Mari had. We hoped to advise people about how to keep their spirits up, as Andrea did. And we were both interested in researching alternative therapies, because we had tried conventional ones such as drugs and surgery but were still in pain. We decided to write this book for the newly diagnosed person because we didn't want others to go through the nightmare that we did. We wanted others to benefit from our experiences. We also wanted to have as much control over our illness as possible.

The idea for this book was originally Mari's. After combing bookstores and libraries for information and not finding enough, Mari put up flyers in local stores, newspapers, and her doctor's office, looking for people who wanted to be interviewed about their experiences. Andrea saw the flier, wrote down the number, and then promptly forgot about it for two months until she happened to see it again in her journal. At the time the two met to do the interview, Mari's editorial partner had become ill and had to bow out of the project. Andrea stepped in to do the job.

During the interview process, patients were given a questionnaire (reproduced below) as a guideline for discussion. Interviews were conducted either in person or over the telephone. Many people mentioned the names of doctors and other treatment providers who had been helpful to them. Some of those practitioners contributed articles to this book. While many of the providers we interviewed are located in Seattle, Washington (because that's where we live), we have included an extensive Resources guide at the back of the book that gives readers information about treatment providers all across the United States.

This book explores various treatment alternatives for FM and CFS. Each chapter focuses on a different alternative; in most chapters, the reader hears first from a treatment provider and then reads an interview with a person who has dealt with that subject personally. We have included information on acupuncture, massage therapy, and Chinese remedies, narcotics (including the controversial use of medical marijuana for pain and muscle spasm), and movement and physical therapies, as well as an overview of the more traditional treatments for these conditions. Advice on legal matters and obtaining Social Security and private disability benefits is also included. The latest research and fundraising is discussed. Twenty-eight care providers, teachers, and attorneys have contributed to this book.

Through these interviews with patients and providers, we hope that the reader will obtain a thorough knowledge of FM and CFS and the range of techniques that can be used to treat them. We've also included an extensive bibliography at the back of the book to give readers a way to research the topic for themselves.

Given our cognitive difficulties and physical limitations, writing this book has been a real labor of love for us. It's more than a little ironic that tragedy is what brought us together, and what brought this project to life. We wanted to learn more about our illnesses, to help others, and to educate them about their options. Before we wrote this book, we were both having a hard time coming to terms with our situation. We both felt that we had a hole in our lives that we were unable to fill despite the therapies, the support groups, the love of our families and friends. Writing this book has given us the means to reclaim the sense of purpose and place in the world we lost when we became ill.

And so this project became more than just a publishing contract for us. It literally threw us a lifeline and gave us a reason to get up in the morning, a reason to find a better quality of life for ourselves despite the pain. It gave us back some control over the illness that has controlled our lives for so long. The very fact that this book exists is living proof that people with chronic illness can set goals, have dreams, and accomplish what they want. It just takes a greater commitment, and more time, than it does other people. And yes, we hurt more, but the payoff is well worth the added pain.

This is the challenge for injured people everywhere. We've been forced to find new ways of doing things, of allocating our energies so that we are still able to do what we enjoy. Pacing oneself is a valuable skill to learn. How can you write a book about how difficult it is to live with chronic pain and fatigue while you're living in chronic pain and fatigue? You do it one paragraph, one page, one idea at a time.

Every day that passes brings new research, new information, and new hope for treating FM and CFS. More people are learning about how to manage their chronic pain and fatigue. Attitudes are changing, too: CFS is no longer the "yuppie flu." FM is no longer "just in our heads." Eventually, there may even be a cure. Until that time, education is vitally important. FM patient Sharon W. put it this way: "Coping is just a matter of finding out as much information as I can."

This book is dedicated to those brave souls who went before us down the path of FM and CFS, who found out through tedious trial and error what does and does not make the pain a little more bearable. This book includes the options and information that took many of us years to find on our own. We hope that this book will prevent you, the reader, from facing the sorts of problems and roadblocks that many of us have encountered along the way. And we hope that through reading these incredible stories you will realize that you are not alone. There is still significant debate about the origins of FM and CFS, and still no cure for either syndrome. But we survivors have learned a few secrets along the way, and we're glad to share our tips for getting the most out of life.

We hope this book makes as much of a difference in your life as it has in ours. In return, we ask only that you keep an open mind and are willing to join us in our adventures in healing.

▪ The Questionnaire

The following list of questions is the one used during interviews with patients and providers.

Diagnosis

1. When were you diagnosed, and what made you see a doctor?

2. How long had you been ill prior to your diagnosis?

3. Was it difficult to get a diagnosis of FM or CFS?

4. Prior to your illness, did you have any exposure to chemicals or pesticides, traumas (either physical or mental), accidents, surgeries, or viral illnesses?

5. Do you have any other illness or condition commonly associated with FM or CFS, such as temporomandibular joint disorder or irritable bowel syndrome?

6. How did you feel when you were first told you had FM or CFS?

7. What was your life like before FM and CFS?

Treatment

8. What sort of medications do you take, and what other therapies have you tried?

9. Did they help?

10. How has your lifestyle changed since your diagnosis?

Living with FM and CFS

11. How do you cope with having FM and/or CFS?

12. What is your support network like?

13. Did you lose your job? If so, what was that like?

14. Are you on disability? If so, how long did it take to get disability insurance?

15. Has your illness caused you financial difficulty?

16. How do you deal with the societal pressures on people who are ill?

17. Has being sick changed your life?

18. Has it affected you on a spiritual level?

Chapter 1

The Diagnosis

OBTAINING A DIAGNOSIS of FM or CFS can be a difficult journey. In this chapter, practitioners and patients explain how an accurate diagnosis of these syndromes is obtained. Included here are both technical perspectives from experts in the field and personal anecdotes from people who have sought a diagnosis. Many people have had great difficulty in dealing with uninformed physicians, as the patients interviewed in this chapter reveal. Thus, we hope to persuade readers to be as persistent as possible in pursuing a diagnosis and to gather as much information as they can before embarking on a treatment program. Also included in this chapter is information on diagnosis of a closely related syndrome, myofascial pain syndrome.

Prior to 1990, FM and CFS were consistently misdiagnosed or undiagnosed entirely. Because physicians were either ill-informed on the subject or simply didn't believe that the conditions exist, obtaining an accurate diagnosis was extremely difficult. Only in the last ten years, since the American College of Rheumatology developed an updated "trigger-point" criteria in 1990 as a means of diagnosing FM, has it become easier to get a diagnosis of FM. CFS, too, has gained legitimacy since it was dismissed as "yuppie flu" in the 1980s. Still, there is great dissent among physicians about the causes of FM and CFS. Patients are frequently caught in the crossfire.

Finding the correct treatment can also be a long and complex process. FM and CFS have so many symptoms that physicians often treat patients on a symptom-by-symptom basis rather than realizing that all the symptoms are part of a larger problem. This is one of the reasons that diagnosis is so difficult. This nearsighted approach overlooks the holistic aspects of healing and contributes to our difficulties in finding adequate relief from our pain.

Physicians should suspect FM when the following symptoms occur simultaneously: widespread body pain, fatigue, irritable bowel and bladder, sleep disorders, headaches, and cognitive difficulties (other symptoms may be present as well). For CFS, generalized fatigue lasting six months or more, short-term memory loss and concentration problems, sore throat, tender lymph nodes, sleep disorders, and headaches should clue the doctor in to the presence of this illness. Many CFS patients also report a low-grade fever.

The causes of FM and CFS are not yet fully understood, although there may be a link with physical or emotional trauma. Six of the patients we interviewed for this book developed FM and/or CFS after being injured in an automobile accident. Dr. Mark J. Pellegrino, who wrote *Fibromyalgia: Managing the Pain*, addressed the question of why some people get post-traumatic FM and others exposed to the same trauma do not:

I believe that genetic susceptibility or vulnerability plays a key role…. The vulnerable person may not have any symptoms of FM whatsoever [prior to a trauma], even though the muscles are susceptible to this condition. The susceptible muscles and soft tissues are functioning adequately and are not painful.

Once the soft tissues are traumatized, however, the altered pain responses are triggered and the previous pain-free balance is forever disrupted, resulting in a permanently altered balance that is now painful. The muscles were pushed over the edge, so to speak.

Three women we interviewed, Annie D., Hilary S., and Jody E., were injured while riding in cars that were rear-ended. Jody says, "Sometimes I can't help but wonder how four members of the same family could be in the same car accident but I was the only one diagnosed with FM."

Current research indicates that FM pain, especially in the case of post-traumatic FM, may be caused by the body's overproduction of a neurotransmitter called "Substance P." This neurochemical is associated with the transmission of pain perception to other areas of the body. When the body is injured, Substance P is released into the spinal cord; thus, if Substance P is overproduced, the brain may believe that the body is in more pain than it really is.

Dr. I. Jon Russell, a prominent FM researcher in San Antonio, Texas, tested the cerebrospinal fluid of patients with FM and compared it to that of healthy individuals. Results of testing done in 1994 indicated a higher level of Substance P in people with FM when compared to control individuals. According to Dr. Pellegrino, injured muscle tissues can become chronically painful in some people, even though the initial muscle injury has long since subsided. This could explain why the prevalence of FM is higher among people who have been injured in car accidents.

"When I look back on it now, it seems that I was having some trauma in my life and then maybe the car accident pushed me over the edge," says thirty-four-year-old Becky R., another woman we interviewed for the book. "The car accident was mentally and emotionally traumatic; physically, it was a bad one. I was thrown out of the front windshield and rolled on the ground. I didn't break any bones; I was incredibly fortunate in that respect. I was just bruised, but there was a lot of emotional trauma involved as well."

For Hilary S., a twenty-nine-year-old woman who is now a real-estate agent, life was good before she was hurt in an auto accident. "I was working out three or four times a week. I was full of energy and in really good shape," Hilary says. "I was a happy-go-lucky person. I had lots of friends and was very active, always out doing something or socializing. Months after the accident, I started to have pain. I tired easily. I used to have a photographic memory, but suddenly I realized I didn't remember a thing. I couldn't make words. I started to gain weight quickly. I was irritable all the time. It just progressively got worse."

Andrew M., a forty-six-year-old former electronics technician, said he was diagnosed with FM in 1993, about six months after he had been hit from behind in a car accident. "Some of my symptoms hadn't gone away and were actually getting worse," he says. "I went to see a diagnostician, and he started pressing these places on my body. It felt like I had bruises wherever he touched me. When he finished, he said, 'I think you have fibromyalgia.' I said, 'What in the world is fibromyalgia?' He told me it was a chronic thing that lasts the rest of your life, and that it affects different people on different levels. He sent me to a rheumatologist for a second opinion. It wasn't too difficult to get the diagnosis at that point; the rheumatologist confirmed that I had FM."

Melinda N., a fifty-two-year-old author, said FM symptoms set in within two months of her car accident. Her doctor told her, "You've sprained your back. If it gets better, don't bother to come back." But her condition did not get better; in fact, she began to experience more pain. "The pain was traveling to my shoulder and my neck, and the symptoms were beginning to get very bad," Melinda says. "I had been in good health before, but all of a sudden I was in constant pain. It gradually spread to all parts of my body, everywhere, all the time. I was virtually suicidal, and I still hadn't received any diagnosis. My husband urged me to continue searching for a good doctor. I had thirteen vertebrae out of alignment at once, so the symptoms were full-blown by the time I finally found a doctor who knew what the problem was. It took me four years to get that diagnosis."

Other people we interviewed reported long and difficult searches for a diagnosis, and were greatly relieved when one was finally obtained.

Ellen J., a thirty-eight-year-old social worker, was diagnosed with CFS in 1988 and with FM in 1993. "I was in medical school, but I was in tremendous pain and couldn't sit in class long enough to take notes," Ellen says. "My hands were seizing up, my muscles were spasming from head to toe, my jaw was trembling, I had headaches, and I had to go to the bathroom a lot. After I had seen several doctors who had no idea what was wrong, the dean recommended that I see a rheumatologist. In no time at all, he diagnosed me with FM.

"I was actually relieved when I got the diagnosis," Ellen says. "At first, I thought I had multiple sclerosis, and it was a relief to know I didn't have that. But it was a real bummer, because I was trying to go to medical school, and now I had a really serious condition that wouldn't kill me but was terribly difficult to get over, was not very well understood, and there was no clear treatment for it. Throughout the first couple of years, I had a lot of trouble figuring out what my real capabilities were."

Many other people say that they were relieved to get a diagnosis after years of going from doctor to doctor but not finding out what was making them hurt so badly. But for others, getting the actual diagnosis was in itself a traumatic experience. Nine months after her car accident, Andrea recalls that she sat in the parking lot of her doctor's office, looked at a piece of paper with "post-traumatic FM" written on it, and cried. Anna K. had the same experience. "I remember that after I got home from seeing the doctor," she says, "I just sat and cried. FM is a very chronic and debilitating condition. I couldn't possibly work and carry on my life. I had to change everything."

A lot of patients report thinking that they were going crazy because no one could find what was wrong with them. Sandra W. says, "When I finally got to see my doctor, I said, 'Help me, please, because I'm at the end of my rope.'" Some patients have even had surgery based on inaccurate diagnoses or in an attempt to cure pain that actually came from FM.

One overweight patient reports that her primary care physician told her to "exercise, exercise" after an auto accident. When she replied that any attempt to strenuously exercise brought on "lightning bolts" of pain up and down her legs, the doctor sneered, "You strike me as the kind of person who has no trouble finding excuses not to exercise!" Having FM and CFS is difficult enough without dealing with doctors who have bad attitudes or don't know enough about these syndromes; this only takes away precious energy that could be used for healing.

David A., a thirty-six-year-old who worked in the computer software industry before he became ill, says he too had seen numerous physicians and tried several remedies before he was accurately diagnosed. "I was really worried. I saw a rheumatologist; I went to a neurologist; I tried movement therapy. Then a friend loaned me a book, *Fibromyalgia and Chronic Myofascial Pain Syndrome: A Survival Manual*, by Dr. Devin Starlanyl and Mary Ellen Copeland. I immediately knew that I had FM; there were so many correlations between what I felt and the symptoms discussed in the book.

"I went back to get retested for trigger points, and by that time I had more sensitivity in those areas. So the tests that had originally failed now showed something. With this new knowledge, I could now try therapies that worked for other people. I got all kinds of feedback on things to try, what worked for people and what didn't. And, luckily, FM isn't life-threatening or progressive."

Diane K., too, searched for a diagnosis for a long time. When she first became sick with CFS and FM, she was "working full-time as a special-education teacher *and* teaching aerobics classes *and* teaching sign-language classes," she says. "It was one of those typical overachiever lifestyles. At the time, I was taking antidepressant medications for a panic disorder that developed after my sister died; that, in retrospect, was a post-traumatic stress reaction to her death. It seems to me now that the medication did suppress the panic attacks, and that was great, but then the trauma came out in other ways. I've always believed that the CFS was a manifestation of my beat-up immune system."

At first she thought she had the flu, so she "took the typical few days off, then went back to work. I still felt sick, but I thought it would dwindle in a couple of days. More time went by, and I didn't feel any better. I had a low-grade fever and swollen glands, plus a cough and headaches. I started getting frightened that I had something horribly wrong with me. But I don't think I had cognitive problems at the time (the doctor asked me that, and I said no).

"I started seeing a doctor who mentioned CFS after testing me for everything under the sun twice. I was kind of fortunate that I had a fever, because at least I had some physical proof that I was sick. I know that a lot of people experience disbelief from their doctors, but I had a physical manifestation that convinced them something really was wrong with me. My doctor wanted to test me again, but I was tired of being poked and probed and tested. Finally, I saw a doctor in Beverly Hills, California, who diagnosed me with both CFS and FM. By then, I'd been sick for five or six years, and when he diagnosed me, I cried in his office. I told him, 'God, I feel like such a dork.' But it felt so good to hear somebody say, 'Yes, you have something—it's real!' That's a typical response, he said; he was totally used to hearing it."

Sharon W., who has FM, says, "It started when I was still in high school, the soreness around the joints and overall muscle achiness. The pediatricians thought it was arthritis, which would get a little worse as I got a little older. So I went to see a rheumatologist and found out that I did not have arthritis, I had FM. Luckily, he was educated on it. He gave me all the information he had available at the time, which was only a couple of paper flyers. FM was relatively new then. Nobody wanted to believe it was anything except a mental illness."

The search for an accurate diagnosis often leads people to search for possible causes, as well. Sherry J., a fifty-eight-year-old mother of three, says she is convinced that heredity plays a bigger role in CFS and FM than anyone realizes. "There's a lot of arthritis in my family," she says. "My dad was sick all his life, too. I think he had FM or something like it that no one ever diagnosed. He probably had irritable bowel syndrome, too, and he had his first stroke from a thyroid problem. Now doctors know that thyroid disorders can cause strokes, and they're beginning to find that a lot of people with FM have thyroid disorders. That's what they're battling with me, too. I had my first Cesarean section at eighteen and had three major surgeries after that. I had two bad car accidents prior to the FM diagnosis. I fell asleep at the wheel both times; I never knew I had a sleep disorder.

Two of my three children have these problems, too. I wasn't at all surprised when my daughter was diagnosed with FM."

If you suspect you have FM or CFS, you must be persistent about getting the medical care you deserve. Achieving the best level of health we can depends upon finding qualified people to treat our illnesses. You are ultimately responsible for your health and well-being, and the first step to feeling better is empowering yourself to take control of your healing. There are many skilled, compassionate physicians who are able to correctly diagnose and treat these problems. The Arthritis Foundation can provide a list of rheumatologists in your area (see the Resources section at the back of this book).

Remember, though, that if a doctor tells you that the pain is all in your head, it's time to find another doctor. When you search for a doctor, make sure you ask the following questions:

1. Do you believe that FM and CFS exist?

2. Are you willing to be a partner with me in my healing?

3. If I want to try a different or alternative healing technique, are you willing to keep an open mind and listen to me?

One way to find out about a prospective doctor's treatment approach is to schedule an interview and then ask the questions above. Scheduling a fifteen-minute interview with any prospective doctor is a good way to avoid heartache later. Too many people fail to question their physicians. Remember that the doctor works for you, not the other way around.

While this chapter deals predominantly with the process of obtaining an accurate diagnosis, the providers featured in this section also discuss some conventional treatment plans that should be considered once the diagnosis has been made. For more information on these options, please refer to Chapter 3.

Formal Diagnosis & Treatment of Fibromyalgia

Dr. Philip Mease

Dr. Philip Mease is a rheumatologist in private practice in Seattle. He is also a clinical associate at the University of Washington and is the director of clinical research at Minor & James Medical. He also writes and lectures on the subjects of rheumatology and FM, and is a medical consultant for the Center for Comprehensive Care, a clinic that includes physical therapists, counselors, acupuncturists, occupational therapists, nurses, and biofeedback therapists.

The formal definition of FM, according to the American College of Rheumatology, is very simple: a history of chronic, generalized aching and the finding, during a physical exam, of at least eleven out of eighteen of the so-called tender points." Tender points, when pressed, are more tender than other points in the body; why these specific eighteen sites are more tender, we still don't know, but these seem to be consistently painful in examinations by physicians who consider themselves experts in the field.

Other symptoms often present in someone with FM include fatigue, sleep disturbance, headache, and irritable bowel syndrome (characterized by crampy abdominal pain and either constipation or diarrhea, alternating with normal bowel function). Symptoms also include irritable bladder syndrome, known as interstitial cystitis, a condition in which a person has frequent or painful urination, without any evidence of infection in the urine. Although these are some of the major accompanying signs and symptoms that can be present in someone with FM, they are not a formal part of the definition of the condition.

FM can be present on its own—without any other diagnosis being made—or it can accompany another condition. Often, another chronic pain condition such as degenerative arthritis, rheumatoid arthritis, lupus, or other chronic musculoskeletal pain problems is present. FM can be seen in conjunction with endocrine conditions, thyroid problems, infectious diseases, or Lyme disease. Often, FM arrives in someone who is physically or emotionally stressed; for example, it can also occur in someone with depression who is undergoing stress, such as the stress caused by a difficult divorce.

It's also been widely noted that people with FM have disturbances in various phases of sleep, particularly the deepest, most restorative phase of sleep. There is some correlation between an off-kilter nervous system and disturbances in this phase of sleep. Thus, if doctors and FM patients work toward restoring normal sleep physiology, they can often achieve improvement in the pain levels that patients experience.

Once a diagnosis has been made, treatment programs should be implemented as soon as possible. Certain medications have proven very helpful for many people. A combination that I often use to treat this problem is a small dose of Trazodone, an antidepressant, at bedtime, and a small dose of either Paxil or Zoloft (antidepressants) in the morning. Paxil helps fatigue and pain; Zoloft helps sleep disturbance and pain. Many other medicines can work, either alone or in combination, including the older tricyclic antidepressants such as amitriptyline, Doxepin, or nortriptyline (these can be used at bedtime); Prozac or another nonsedating medicine such as Wellbutrin or Serzone can be used during the day. Doctors can use very, very small doses of these antidepressants, much smaller than you would think could have any effect on depression, and often they'll see a significant improvement in sleep and pain.

Anti-inflammatory medicines, such as ibuprofen or naproxen, can also be used. Sometimes they seem to help; sometimes they don't work at all. It's certainly fair for people to try them. We may briefly use Robaxin, Soma, Flexeril, or other muscle relaxants for short-term pain reduction, but we don't tend to use those on a long-term basis; a good time to use them is when a person has a flare-up of pain. We certainly try to avoid narcotics, because they could lead to dependence by the person who uses them. There are a number of other medicines that can be used; you can find more about them on my Web page [see the Notes on Contributors section].

Some physicians choose another approach, tender-point injections. This involves injecting a numbing agent, either Lidocaine or Procaine, into the body's tender points. (We tend to avoid injecting steroids into these areas if we can because they could cause atrophy of the skin or muscle.) Some physicians prefer the tender-point injection method, but I don't use it, because my general feeling is that its benefits are only temporary. Other doctors may choose to make an injection only if there is an especially painful tender point.

It's also important to treat the individual symptoms of FM, such as irritable bowel syndrome, irritable bladder syndrome, and headaches. Specific approaches can be taken here. For treating irritable bowel and bladder syndromes, a popular medicine is Levsinex, a smooth-muscle relaxant. For irritable bowel symptoms, we also recommend a high-fiber diet and Bentyl, which is an antispasmodic.

My clinic has developed a multidisciplinary treatment program for patients with FM and CFS. We have found that we get much better results by approaching treatment in a multidisciplinary way, using many nonmedication techniques that are useful for the patients. Thus, after their medical diagnoses and management are underway, patients work either individually or in a group with various therapists in our facility.

One technique that we use is stretching. Another is generalized aerobic conditioning: swimming, using a Stairmaster, walking on the treadmill; anything that gets your heart rate up and makes you break a sweat tends to be good for FM. Other techniques are hands-on therapy, such as myofascial release (a stretching technique) that's done by a physical therapist or a massage therapist. Also, acupuncture can be helpful for some patients, as can various forms of meditation—simple meditation, relaxation, biofeedback, or movement therapy in the form of *tai chi*. At my clinic, we've developed *tai chi* classes specifically for people with FM and CFS.

We also try to treat accompanying conditions that may stimulate or aggravate FM. I mentioned earlier that accompanying degenerative arthritis, rheumatoid arthritis, lupus, or thyroid problems can all contribute to the presence of FM, so it's appropriate to address these conditions independently to make sure that all of them are adequately treated. The reasoning behind this is that if we decrease pain symptoms or other aspects of accompanying illnesses, we can lessen the FM stimulus itself.

Another important aspect of treatment is development of an emotional support system. Once a diagnosis is made, it's very important for the patient to have people to talk to, someone to empathize with them and be supportive. Family members, spouses, boyfriends or girlfriends, relatives, friends, support groups, therapy groups of various kinds, friends at the swimming pool or at church—this kind of human exchange is a vital part of the care of a person with any chronic illness.

A Patient's Story: Ann A.

Ann is forty-six years old and has a degree in environmental health. She worked in occupational health and safety for seven years, during which time she was exposed to harmful chemicals. After leaving the job, she went back to school to study accounting. She was an accountant for twelve years before she became too ill with FM to continue working.

I was diagnosed in January of 1994, but it took almost a year to get to that point. In early 1993, what I call my "acute" phase of FM started. I was having lower-back pain and pain in my hips.

I went to my regular physician many times, but she thought I'd just strained my back or something. We tried some anti-inflammatories for a while; that didn't work. And eventually I started having substantial tailbone pain. My doctor said, "Well maybe you just fell on it," and I said, "No, I didn't fall!" I knew I hadn't done anything to aggravate it specifically.

After several months of trying assorted things—mostly anti-inflammatories and ice—and my condition not changing, my doctor decided to do an X-ray. Of course, the X-ray showed nothing. I was becoming really adamant and not very nice about the fact that I had this horrendous pain and couldn't even sit. She finally sent me to an orthopedist, who injected cortisone into my tailbone. But even that only gave me a little relief for a short while, so the doctor said, "Well, we'll do it a second time. After that, we may want to consider surgery." I said, "No way…. No one is going to lop off my tailbone!"

The orthopedist thought maybe I was just out of condition and needed to strengthen the muscles around the hips. He sent me to a physical therapist, but I didn't respond to treatment at all. But this therapist was the one who said, "I think there's something else going on here. You need to see a good diagnostician." She recommended another doctor, who finall~

He handed me a littl~ Foundation and said, "The good news ~ad news is, it can be a long, drawn-ou~ ~scomfort." And you know what doctor~ ~e told me that one treatment is low doses of antidepressants, and sent me on my way with a prescription and this pamphlet. I walked out the door in shock. I'd just been told I had this chronic, long-term pain syndrome, and I was kind of numb.

Prior to my diagnosis, I had had several traumatic events in my life: I divorced, my mother died suddenly, and I broke up with my business partner of ten years. Those stresses were part of bringing myself into the acute phase of FM; I think that a series of "insults" to my body caused the FM. That's one theory of why we develop it; for some reason, some people have a genetic predisposition to it. We're not able to handle certain stresses, and when we experience them, they are the straw that breaks the camel's back.

In hindsight, I know that the FM had probably been going on for about ten years. I had had a long series of physical problems. When he gave me the diagnosis, my doctor told me I was lucky not to have lost any more of my body than I already had. Imagine, I had eight surgeries in eight years. In 1982, I had TMJ [temporomandibular joint disorder] surgery to realign my lower jaw. In 1984, I had a bunionectomy on my left foot to removed extra bone growth (I had so much pain prior to that surgery that I could barely find shoes to wear). In 1986, I had a bunionectomy on my right foot. In 1987, I had arthro-

21

scopic surgery on the TMJ. In 1988, I had a total hysterectomy (which I opted for when painful menstrual cycles made me almost nonfunctional two weeks per month). In 1990, I had two bowel obstruction surgeries. The obstructions were scar tissue formed as a result of the endometriosis and the hysterectomy. That same year, I had a second arthroscopic surgery on the TMJ.

The multiple surgeries show how the doctors were chasing the pain I felt in various parts of my body. That's characteristic of many doctors: When you're having pain, they either want to give you drugs or operate on you, because those are their only options when they don't know what's going on. If I could do it all over again, knowing what I now know, I would never go through all those surgeries. I thought that I had to in order to feel better, but the surgeries actually made me worse.

I experienced acute, continuous FM symptoms for the next four years. In 1994, I received the diagnosis of FM and had to quit work. Soon after I was first diagnosed, I went into counseling. My counselor and I used the metaphor of severely pruning a tree. I had cut back to the core, the utter essence. Being ill forces you to shift priorities and let go of what you used to think was important. But after every pruning, there's new growth. FM has forced me to adopt a different lifestyle, but I think it's a lifestyle that's much healthier than the way a lot of people live—sort of mindlessly. FM has distilled my life down to what's really important.

Fibromyalgia and Myofascial Pain Syndrome

Dr. Devin Starlanyl

Dr. Devin Starlanyl is author of *The Fibromyalgia Advocate: Getting the Support You Need to Cope with Fibromyalgia and Myofascial Pain Syndrome.* She is also coauthor of *Fibromyalgia and Chronic Myofascial Pain Syndrome: A Survival Manual.*

Myofascial pain syndrome is often confused with FM, and people may have both conditions at the same time. FM and myofascial pain syndrome are two of the three most common causes of chronic pain (the third is joint dysfunction). Both are frequently misdiagnosed, and are often undiagnosed entirely. Usually, the patient goes through about ten doctors and spends ten years or longer just getting a diagnosis, and often patients are given many inappropriate therapies along the way. Sometimes the patient even becomes totally disabled during that time.

Chronic myofascial pain syndrome is a condition of body-wide trigger points that are maintained by perpetuating factors, such as lack of sleep or poor sleep position.

Most of us have seen the white translucent covering on the muscles of chicken we buy at the grocery store. That is myofascia. This sticky covering wraps around bundles of muscle cells and around the muscles themselves. It interconnects throughout the whole body. Myofascia is very sticky stuff; it sticks together to form tendons and ligaments at the ends of muscles. When the body experiences pain, the myofascia responds: the body reacts to pain immediately (because pain signifies damage), and the body goes into a self-protective stress mode. When this happens, the myofascia forms a sort of "splint," trying to minimize the pain by restricting movement. This "guarding" is part of the body's survival mechanism and is helpful on a short-term basis.

But when pain becomes chronic and guarding lasts, the muscle tightness inhibits the delivery of fuel and oxygen, as well as removal of waste. An area of extreme sensitivity can develop. This is called a myofascial trigger point, and it is an area that is very painful when pressed and can refer pain and other symptoms in specific patterns throughout the body. When a muscle has trigger points, it becomes weakened and shorter and cannot stretch or do its normal job. It loses range of motion. Myofascial trigger points are not the same as the "tender points" found in FM patients [see the Foreword for a discussion of tender points], but they are neuromuscular in nature.

In myofascial pain syndrome, the muscle becomes hard as rock. Often the trigger points can't be felt because of fluid in the muscles. Everything is very, very tight, and people may feel like they are wearing a wet suit that is several sizes too small. Even the tightness itself can be painful.

Anyone can develop a myofascial trigger point, but if there are no perpetuating factors, it will become latent and won't cause symptoms unless it's activated (and if properly treated, it will go away). Perpetuating factors can include lack of sleep, pain, or certain body movements or positions. Even a poor sleeping position can be a perpetuating condition. Because these problems often accompany FM, people with FM are at special risk of developing myofascial pain syndrome. Although myofascial pain syndrome is not a progressive disorder, if you have a perpetuating factor such as FM and the trigger points are untreated or improperly treated, your body will soon develop a network of nodules and ropy bands.

Trigger points tend to breed other trigger points. When a muscle is weakened by trigger points, another muscle will try to overcompensate. The overworked muscle then develops trigger points, which are called secondary trigger points. Trigger points also develop in muscles inside the referred pain pattern. These are called satellite trigger points.

When a person with FM develops a trigger point, it will quickly lead to secondary and satellite trigger points, and the patient can develop myofascial pain syndrome unless the trigger point is properly and immediately treated. Myofascial pain syndrome may exist head-to-toe in some people, but the syndrome is made up of individual, overlapping trigger-point referral patterns. There may be a trigger point in the middle of a referral pattern, on the side of the pattern, or even outside the pattern. Each trigger point has a specific pain pattern, which is recognizable from patient to patient.

Diagnosing trigger points is a problem only if the doctor is not familiar with specific trigger-point referral patterns. The situation may be further complicated if the patient has symptoms other than pain that are caused by the trigger points. For example, trigger points can cause dizziness, cause the knees or ankles to give out, or cause people to drop things. People may stagger and walk into walls, or their vision may blur. There are a lot of other bizarre symptoms that can come with trigger points—such as the inability to perceive the amount of weight you have in your hand. This will cause you to drop things and lose control. All of these symptoms may make getting a correct diagnosis more difficult.

People with FM may suffer from sleep disorders, which can be perpetuating factors contributing to the development of myofascial pain syndrome. When the body and the brain talk to each other, they use neurotransmitters and other informational substances (electrobiochemicals that transport messages between the brain and body). In the case of FM, these neurochemicals don't work properly and get out of balance. This starts a neurotransmitter cascade, because every neurotransmitter is balanced by another in the body, and hormones and other important biochemicals are regulated by neurotransmitters. Neurotransmitters are regulated in delta sleep, and people with FM don't get enough of this sleep. They are jolted awake or into shallow sleep by the intrusion of alpha waves (awake brain waves), so that they either wake up many times during the night or sleep very shallowly. People wake up feeling like they've been hit by a truck; they ache all over and feel stiff because the cellular repair and neurotransmitter balancing that the body needs hasn't happened.

So sleep deprivation is a major handicap for people with FM, and it is a perpetuating factor that needs to be addressed right away. (Incidentally, sleep deprivation was used in World War II as a form of torture.) Sleep deprivation causes a lot of what we call "fibro fog" and cognitive deficit memory problems. So it's critical for the FM patient to get restorative sleep.

Another problem is that people with FM can get very toxic because they can't get rid of wastes in their bodies. There is growing evidence that certain biochemicals are higher in people with FM, such as hyaluronic acid, quinolinic acid, and phosphoric acid. Many of these substances are irritants. As pollution of the body increases, people become more susceptible to myofascial trigger points.

People who have both FM and myofascial pain syndrome experience different problems from tender points and trigger points. FM's tender points can cause all-over achiness. You can't have FM "in your back" or in your neck or hands. It's like saying you're "a little bit preg-

nant." You either have it all over or you don't. Myofascial trigger points, however, usually cause localized pain. FM also gives you the flu-like feeling that never seems to let up. This fatigue is generally caused by lack of sleep.

When a person has multiple trigger points and a genetic predisposition to FM, it appears that FM will develop unless both conditions are promptly treated. When FM and myofascial pain syndrome occur in the same patient, it can be more than double trouble. In FM, the nervous system is like a stereo stuck on high. Every sensation becomes intensified, including the pain, dizziness, and other sensations caused by the trigger points of the myofascial pain syndrome. To break this cycle, you must identify all perpetuating factors and treat them vigorously.

FM and myofascial trigger points require different treatments, even when they coexist in the same patient. One of the more unusual therapies, which seems to work in a large percentage of people with FM, is guaifenesin, an expectorant that's often found in cough syrup. Guaifenesin can help the body remove waste matter from the muscles. Use of this medication in FM patients was pioneered by Dr. R. Paul St. Amand, an endocrinologist in Marina del Rey, California. But guaifenesin dosage is very specific to the patient and can easily be blocked, so the treatment protocol is very specific. You cannot just go out and take cough medicine and expect to reverse FM. For more information, you might consult the guaifenesin support group on the Internet [see Resources].

To properly treat myofascial pain syndrome, you should find a good stretching program and learn a variety of physical therapies. Many techniques can be helpful; often chiropractic and massage therapy can be a big help. Breathing, too, is very important. Make sure you breathe properly—avoid paradoxical or shallow chest breathing, which can perpetuate trigger points and make you oxygen starved. You need to "belly" breathe: When you breathe in, your belly should come out. You should also do mind work as well as body work, because your mental state is very important.

Your body habits count a lot, too. If you smoke, you must decide whether you want to keep smoking or get rid of your trigger points, because it is almost impossible to successfully treat trigger points if you continue to smoke. You can also attack these conditions by detoxifying your life as much as possible. Develop a good diet—avoid processed food and find a healthy balance between foods, such as the "Zone" diet. Many patients are sensitive to carbohydrates, and the diet today is overwhelmingly carbohydrate-heavy. Deficiencies of certain vitamins and minerals, such as B1, B6, B12, folic acid, and magnesium, can be major perpetuating factors.

There are many ways to work on perpetuating factors. Luckily, you can do a lot of these things yourself. FM and myofascial pain syndrome are time-consuming conditions, but your goals should focus on self-maintenance and returning to function and the highest possible quality of life. Although there is currently no cure for FM, many of its symptoms can be reversed. Myofascial trigger points, too, can be reversed by identifying and thoroughly dealing with perpetuating factors. You can improve your life situation and function very well, and many techniques are available. You just have to find the combination that works for you.

■ A Patient's Story: Tom O.

Tom O. is forty-six years old and works for a Northwest telephone company. He's been married for twenty-six years and has two children. His family lives in Renton, Washington, and despite his illness he intends to continue working as long as he can.

It all started back in 1992. I just felt like hell all the time, like somebody stuck me in a sack, threw me down, and walked on my body. All my joints hurt, all my muscles hurt, tendons, ligaments; everything hurt. I'm a lineman for a telephone company, which means a lot of climbing poles, fixing poles, replacing poles, wiring buildings as they're being constructed so that people can have telephone service. It's heavy, physical work. I thought maybe that had something to do with it. I was tired, tired of it all.

27

So I went to my family doctor, but it took a long time to come up with the diagnosis of FM, almost two years. I went back two or three times to tell him that what he'd given me wasn't helping me; there was still something wrong, more than just the regular pain of getting up every day. It's frustrating—sometimes you pay for all these fancy expensive tests and they come back normal. And yet you know there's something going on.

I eventually read an article about FM and asked my doctor, "Do I have FM?" He said, "You're a strong candidate for it." They did more tests on the tender places, and he said, "We're about 112 percent positive that's what it is."

I didn't know a heck of a lot about it before I got diagnosed. I thought, Well, fine, they know what it is now. (How naive I was.) It didn't really shock me. I thought, I can deal with this. I had been dealing with it for a year or two before I even knew what it was. The only difference was that now I had a name for it.

Before I started having symptoms, I had one epileptic seizure, out of nowhere, back in 1989. I got called out to check on a pole that was damaged in a car accident, but I didn't see it. So I came back home and went back to bed. I woke up the next morning about 7 A.M. and two medics were standing over my bed. I'd literally peed all over myself. I'd also chewed my tongue up, and they were looking at me like I'd just grown a third eye. It was quite a wild deal. I couldn't drive for six months. I didn't correlate the seizure with anything at the time, but maybe it did have something to do with the FM. Maybe my brain has a glitch in it that's making everything hurt. I don't know.

I once could do anything, any time, all day long, and not hurt. Baseball, football, hiking, walking, fishing, lifting, pushing, shoving, anything, it didn't matter. Wrestle around with the kids. I could cut firewood all day, stack it, then get up the next day and everything would be just hunky dory. But those days are very rare now. I'm not as quick as I used to be, not as flexible. I've given up playing baseball. I couldn't play as well as I wanted to play and I'm not going to be some old geezer out there and embarrass myself. The thing I probably enjoy the most in life, other than my kids, is hiking, backpacking, going off for a week. Used to be, every other week I'd be gone, just me by myself. That's where I liked it, away from everybody. But I'm getting to the point where I don't know if I can do it any more. It's beginning to wear me down. Last year, I took my youngest brother and kids with me, and I had such a hell of a time that they ended up carrying some of my stuff back. That had never happened before.

My family is my only real support group. My kids are very understanding, luckily. And so is my youngest brother. I've disappointed him once or twice when we've been all set to go on a hike, and then I felt extremely bad and had to call it off. Being diagnosed with a chronic illness is depressing. I'm beginning to wonder, Is this ever going to get better? Maybe I should quit my job, but I can't look anywhere else to earn the money I do now. Luckily, this hasn't affected my marriage. I just moan a little more, and she says, "Yeah, I know." She's always been less physically active than me, so I guess I'm finally slowing down to her speed.

I try to ignore the pain as much as I can. I take a multivitamin every day, but nothing else. (I've never really done any research into anything else to take.) I've always watched what I eat; I try to not eat a lot of fats and meats. I'm only forty-six. I don't want to be an invalid; there's so much to do out there. I don't want to sit back and watch it all go by, as so many people have to do or choose to do. I've never even told my friends about it. These are people I work with. They're a bunch of pretty hardy guys, even though they're old guys, my age and older, so they've all got aches and pains, too. I'm just another worker. I don't want to stick out.

I really wonder, though, if they would understand. I think part of it is that macho-man image thing. If I said, "Hey man, I've got FM and I'm feeling like hell today," maybe they would look at me like, Huh? Women can call up their friends, have a little get-together, and talk about this stuff. "What do you do and how do you get help and blah blah blah." I envy that about women. For a man, though, it's different. We all complain. But we don't really talk about it. We just go on.

I'm a firm believer that if the spirit is willing, the body is able. But, boy, I tell you, the older I get, the more this stuff just doesn't go away. I try not to give up, but it's slowly chipping away at my life, one molecule at a time. Some days I'm just plain physically immobilized. I keep thinking, Well, out of the whole damn encyclopedia of bad things that could happen, this ain't nothin'. Every day, I try to convince myself that this ain't nothin'. Which it isn't, nothing other than one big pain.

Formal Diagnosis and Treatment of Chronic Fatigue Syndrome

Dr. Dedra Buchwald

Dr. Dedra Buchwald is the director of the University of Washington Chronic Fatigue Clinic at Harborview Medical Center in Seattle. She is also the director of the CFS Cooperative Research Center at Harborview.

Chronic fatigue syndrome is a specific illness characterized by severe, persistent fatigue, often associated with difficulties of sleep and concentration, aching muscles and joints, headaches, sore throats, and depression. In clinical populations, it is most commonly diagnosed in previously healthy women between the ages of twenty and fifty, but it can afflict people of all ages and socioeconomic groups.

Most commonly, CFS takes the form of a chronic, recurring, "flu-like" illness; for most patients, some degree of fatigue is present every day. Virtually all patients perceive themselves to be impaired in some way, some severely so. They find that the fatigue, difficulty in concentrating, and pain limit their ability to participate fully in normal life activities. Many patients are depressed or anxious, but generally they feel that the depression and anxiety have followed and been caused by the illness.

There is no single test and no simple way to make the diagnosis of CFS. The diagnosis is usually made based on symptoms alone. On physical examination, an inflamed throat along with swollen lymph glands in the back of the neck and under the armpit may occasionally be seen. More common are points on the muscles that are very sore and tender when pressure is applied.

However, symptoms that are typical of CFS may be caused by other problems, such as thyroid trouble, anemia, infection, or depression. Therefore, the doctor needs to be sure that a patient with symptoms of chronic fatigue does not have one of these conditions, which are far more common than CFS. CFS can only be considered after other causes of chronic fatigue have been excluded.

CFS is characterized by a number of different clinical and laboratory features, all of which can wax and wane over time. Laboratory tests are usually normal. Liver function tests may be slightly elevated. Tests that determine the presence of human herpes virus 6 (HHV6) or Epstein-Barr virus are sometimes abnormal.

To correctly diagnose a person with CFS, physicians should use the criteria developed in 1994 by international consensus at the Centers for Disease Control. To be diagnosed with CFS, a person must meet all of the fatigue criteria listed below, and other conditions must be ruled out. In addition, four out of the eight symptom criteria must be present.

Fatigue Criteria

The fatigue must

1. be of at least six months' duration;

2. not be lifelong (i.e., the person can't remember ever feeling normal);

3. result in a substantial reduction of occupational, educational, social, or personal activities, as compared to the person's activities before the onset of illness;

4. not be the result of ongoing exertion or be relieved by rest.

Symptom Criteria

Symptoms must have started at the same time or after the onset of fatigue, and must be present simultaneously for at least six months during the illness. Patients must meet at least four of these criteria:

1. impairment of short-term memory or concentration that is severe enough to cause a substantial reduction in previous levels of occupational, educational, social, or personal activities

2. sore throat

3. tender lymph nodes in the neck or armpits

4. muscle pain

5. joint pain involving more than one joint, without swelling or redness

6. headaches of a new type, pattern, or severity

7. unrefreshing sleep

8. malaise or fatigue lasting more than twenty-four hours after exertion

Exclusionary Criteria

1. any other medical condition that could mimic CFS—such as a history of malignancy, chronic infection, neuromuscular disease, etc.

2. bipolar affective disorders, psychotic or melancholic depression, schizophrenia, and dementia

3. anorexia nervosa and bulimia

4. alcohol or substance abuse within two years of the onset of fatigue or at any time thereafter

5. severe obesity

CFS probably does not have just one cause; instead, there are many contributing factors [see Rich Carson's article in Chapter 12 for the latest research on possible causes]. Most likely, a large number of triggers cause small changes in the body's immune system, sleep, and hormone production. In CFS patients, these changes are not properly regulated, resulting in the symptoms of CFS. Triggers for CFS may include stress, infections, surgery, depression, physical or emotional abuse, and environmental exposures. What is important is that long after the trigger is gone, the illness continues.

There is no proven connection between CFS and the development of any other serious medical disorder, such as multiple sclerosis or cancer, but several illnesses similar to CFS have been described in medical journals for at least 100 years. One is called neurocirculatory asthenia, which consists of nervous and circulatory system disturbances characterized by fatigue and pain. It is seldom written about in modern medical literature. Another, myalgic encephalomyelitis, has often been described as occurring in small outbreaks and, clinically, is very much like CFS. A third condition, fibromyalgia, is characterized by muscle pain and many tender points on the muscles.

Since the cause of CFS is not known, there are no specific treatments for it. However, a large number of medications have been tried, with varying degrees of success. These include anti-inflammatory agents, antiviral and immunologically active drugs, and low doses of antidepressants. The most widely used treatments are combinations of low doses of serotonin reuptake inhibitors in the morning for energy, and tricyclics in the evening to promote sleep. Patients are also advised to get sufficient sleep and engage in a daily, low-level exercise program—with the assistance of a physical therapist. Cognitive behavioral therapy has proved effective in several clinical trials, and many patients are better able to cope with the illness with the help of a knowledgeable mental-health counselor. Acupuncture, massage therapy, biofeedback, and other nonpharmacological approaches have also provided benefit to some patients. Often, finding an effective treatment is a matter of trial and error. Treatment must be individualized and focused on reducing symptoms.

Although the course of CFS varies greatly, most patients do improve. Up to two-thirds of patients have moderate to complete recovery over the course of several years, though most continue to have some symptoms. Improvement is usually broken by relapses brought on by overexertion, stress, or infection. Only a small percentage of patients experience progressive worsening of their illness.

■ A Patient's Story: Karin L.

Karin is thirty-two years old and lives in Seattle, Washington. She is currently enrolled in graduate school on a part-time basis. In her spare time, she enjoys gardening and weaving.

I received my diagnosis of CFS in the spring of 1991. I had been sick for several months at that point and had been going to the doctor, trying to find out what was going on. Finally, my doctor referred me to an infectious disease specialist. He was known to be a very good diagnostician, and he was the first one who suggested CFS.

My mom made an appointment with a gastroenterologist, because I had had my appendix out right before I got sick. The gastroenterologist first tried to tell me it was all in my head, and he made me take a psychological test. He also did some extensive testing of my gastrointestinal system, and everything came out normal. But he did finally confirm the diagnosis of CFS. At that point, they called it "postviral fatigue syndrome," because I hadn't been sick for six months yet.

I was experiencing a lot of stress about school at the time that I got sick. I was twenty-three, and it was my last year in college. I wasn't sure what I wanted to do. I thought about going into the Peace Corps.

When I first got sick, I thought I was coming down with the flu. The Student Health Center staff were concerned that I had some sort of infection. I didn't get any worse, but I didn't get any better, and I've never felt the same since. I continue to have a sore throat, tender lymph nodes, headache, and low-grade fever. But now my main symptom is the fatigue.

I used to take immune globulin once a week, which seemed to help with some of these symptoms. Now there's a national shortage because of the explosion of hepatitis cases in this country—the one thing that seemed to help and I can't even get it anymore.

In a way, I was relieved when I got the diagnosis, because there was a name for my problem and we finally had an idea of what was happening. But I didn't know anyone else who had CFS, and I had never heard of it until I got sick. I was really scared, because I had read an article about it that listed all sorts of bizarre symptoms. Both doctors told me that I would be well within six to ten months. So I thought, Great, I'll just take it easy. Well, that was seven years ago.

Before I got sick, I was your basic overachiever. I had very good grades; I was active; I liked to run, play soccer, swim, and ski. I had just bought my own car, but until that time I had always used my bike for transportation. The year before, I had traveled in Germany with a backpack, taking the train and doing a lot of walking. I do basically none of those things any more, except for a bit of walking.

Now exercise makes me feel worse (although I have a stretching routine that I try to do). Yesterday, for example, I walked to a video store about three blocks from my house. On the way there, I felt just fine, but about halfway back, I started to feel really tired. It's not the physical exercise alone that causes problems, but in combination with whatever else is going on in my life, that can cause a flare-up in my symptoms. There's "X" amount of energy, and I could spend it all in one place and do a little bit more exercise, but that would mean I spend less time doing social things with people whom I enjoy.

I also meditate. About a year and a half ago, I did a workshop on stress reduction (these programs are starting to spring up all over the country). It helped me to slow me down and relax, which I have found very helpful. Otherwise, I just take one day at a time and rest as much as I can. I really try to honor my body's limits. I've learned that pushing it doesn't help and may make me feel worse. I may get to do more today, but I'll pay for it tomorrow.

I have worked very hard to return to a normal life. I have just finished my first term of graduate school, which I am thoroughly enjoying. It is important to note, however, how I've handled my life to be able to go back to school. I've been lucky; I have a volunteer who comes over once a week and cleans for me, and occasionally does some grocery shopping and other errands.

I'm fortunate to be attending a university that is willing to accommodate my needs. My classes were scheduled in the late afternoon and evening. On class days, I frequently rested in bed until it was time to get ready to leave. I was able to read about half of the materials before the term started. On several written assignments, I was able to demonstrate my learning without having to spend my energy writing final essays. During this time, however, I had virtually no social life outside of school, because I simply had no energy left over. Now I'm planning to cut back on my class load and rebalance my life.

It's a full-time job to be a disabled or chronically ill person. Society really pressures you to work, to provide for yourself, to go and do. Our culture is based on how much you can do, and how much money you make. When you can't do much of anything, it's not easy.

Being sick has changed my life in every imaginable way. I can't do many things that I once enjoyed. But I have found new hobbies, new things I enjoy doing. I've learned the art of lying in bed and doing nothing, which was something I couldn't do very easily before. I've become a lot more conscious of my body, how I'm feeling, and now I'm better about taking care of it.

Chapter 2

Symptoms of Fibromyalgia and Chronic Fatigue Syndrome

I N THIS CHAPTER, we familiarize you with the symptoms of FM and CFS, and offer a few ideas on how managing your symptoms can improve your life and outlook.

If you recognize the following symptoms in yourself, it may be time to take your concerns to your physician. Do you have muscle pain, stiffness, problems falling asleep or staying asleep, constipation alternating with diarrhea, frequent urination, headaches, achiness, difficulty concentrating, depression, or extreme fatigue? If you have a combination of these symptoms, you could be a candidate for a diagnosis of FM. People who have CFS experience sore throats, cognitive difficulties, sleep disturbances, extreme fatigue, cough, low-grade fever, gastrointestinal problems, and sensory dysfunctions. More severe symptoms can include heart palpitations, chest pain, and shortness of breath.

In both syndromes, symptoms range from the mundane to the bizarre. Both CFS and FM can create a situation that we call "filtering." This is a sort of stimulation overload that occurs if there are a lot of stimuli—noise, visual distractions, or smells (such as too much perfume in an elevator). It can cause us to become dizzy, lightheaded, and nauseous. For example, Andrea once went to an electronics store to buy a new television and VCR. Within fifteen minutes, she had become so "foggy" and nauseated that she had to leave the store.

Another unfortunate side effect of these illnesses is severe disorientation. When we're driving, we might suddenly lose our way on a road we've driven every day for ten years. And the more tired we become, the worse it gets. Where is my hat/scarf/shoe/key/paper/phone bill/sanity? Is my appointment at 2 P.M. on the twelfth or 12 P.M. on the second? I've lost my appointment card *again*.

Patients we talked to commented that some of their symptoms—such as hypersensitivity to light and smells—seemed so strange to them that they didn't even mention them to their physicians for fear of being labeled a hypochondriac or mentally unstable. Others mentioned that they were afraid their symptoms were due to a terminal illness such as cancer, and that their pain was going to literally kill them. Still others had a hard time realizing that all their symptoms were part of one condition.

Symptoms of FM and CFS are often confused with those of other conditions, such as multiple sclerosis, lupus, and rheumatoid arthritis. Since too many physicians are still uneducated on the subject, treatment is often on a symptom-by-symptom basis. It's important that you don't attribute each and every symptom to your FM or CFS. Each time a new symptom appears, you must tell your physician about it. One woman said that she had neglected to report a new symptom to her physician, thinking that it was just part of her FM. She later learned that she had terminal cancer.

It is also important to find a physician who does not take your symptoms for granted. If you experience troublesome symptoms and your doctor dismisses them as just part of FM or CFS, it wouldn't hurt to start interviewing new physicians. You may have a problem unrelated to FM or CFS, such as a pinched nerve that causes sciatic pain. The FM or CFS will amplify that pain. If you simply assume that the pain is coming from FM or CFS, then the underlying problem and cause of your pain will go untreated, leading to a vicious cycle of pain. And until that problem is treated, your FM or CFS will continue to be aggravated by it, and vice versa.

Symptoms vary from person to person, and most people experience a number of problems. Tom O., who is a lineman for a telephone company, says that his memory is starting to go—but he'd like to think it's due to age. "Sometimes I'm searching for a word and another word comes out of my mouth. I have a good vocabulary; I'm well read. But some days, I can't pick a word out of the air like I used to. And I get lost when I'm driving more often now. It's part of that whole cognitive thing that's commonly associated with FM.

"Sleep is a real treat, too," he adds. "Most of the time I'm up three or four times a night. That, too, could just be old-age syndrome. I'll go for a month or so where I sleep like a rock. And then, for no reason that I can tell, I'll sleep for two hours and then wake up. Sometimes I lie there for hours before I can get back to sleep. And I don't know if every time I wake up I have to pee, or if I have to pee because I happened to wake up. I've taken amitriptyline, an antidepressant, to help myself sleep.

"I also have the irritable bowel thing; one day it's diarrhea and the next day it's constipation or bloating. Sometimes it will hit me while I'm in the middle of work, and I'm always outdoors where there are no bathrooms."

Dennis H., who has CFS, says that his worst symptom was losing his ability to do physical activity. "During the early years, it was a question of how much rest I needed—several hours of napping in the middle of the day, and I spent most of my time sitting in a chair, reading or watching TV or whatever. But I was always able to get up and around, do what I needed to take care of myself during the day," he says. "I never required anybody to take care of me; I was never bedridden; no one had to bring me food or help with daily activities. My condition wasn't as severe as that of people who have a dramatic onset, in which their health is extremely compromised and they are bedridden or hospitalized.

"As time goes by, I have become more functional; the adverse effects have grown less and less. I can go out and work in the yard or run errands. I don't get as run down, although things do fluctuate. There are good-to-better times, and there are worse times. My symptoms tend to vary depending upon how active I am and the amount of stress and anxiety I'm feeling."

Annie D. has symptoms of both FM and CFS. "My cognitive abilities are scrambled," she says. "I forget things. My awesome vocabulary, in which I once placed so much pride, is now greatly reduced. Words pop out of my mouth in place of the ones I wanted. I get bad headaches. My hands tingle and throb; they feel like they're asleep. I have TMJ [temporomandibular joint disorder], so my jaw pops almost every time I yawn or open my mouth to eat. I am easily nauseated; sometimes even a simple bus ride will put me down for the rest of the week because someone had on too much perfume or had a bad body odor. Combine that with the hard seats, the noise of other bus riders, and the bouncing ride, and it makes for one unhappy behind. I have muscle spasms and pains shooting down my arms, and pain in my hip that runs down the length of my leg. It's a bitch."

Diane K., who also has both CFS and FM, experienced blurred vision, painful skin, and many other symptoms. "The eye doctors really had fun with me, because my vision would go from needing a prescription back to twenty-twenty," Diane says. "The doctors were saying, 'That's impossible! You must have diabetes,' although I was tested over and over again for diabetes. All of a sudden, every one of my symptoms fit into the CFS picture. It was great having one little box to put it all in. Yahoo!"

Ellen J., who has FM and CFS, says, "I have migraine headaches, irritable bowel and bladder, dizziness, temporomandibular joint disorder, cognitive difficulties, fatigue, muscle pain, and aches. I also have multiple chemical sensitivity [MCS], which is a separate diagnosis. One of my doctors told me that 30 percent of people who have FM and/or CFS also meet the diagnostic criteria for MCS. I've had to drastically modify my lifestyle to create a safe environment so that my body can heal. Chemicals that have been identified as triggering reactions include petrochemicals [gasoline, diesel, propane], formaldehyde, paint thinners, resins, pipe and tobacco smoke, perfumes, chemical household cleaners, pesticides, chemical treatments on new clothing, printed materials [solvents in inks], and many other substances. The National Academy of Sciences has estimated that about 15 percent of the population may be affected by environmental illnesses."

Diane's doctor put her on malic acid and Zantac, and she thought she was cured. "For seven months, I didn't have a single symptom. I was walking on clouds, I was so happy. I figured I was cured, so I stopped taking the stuff—and boom, I had a huge relapse. I frantically started taking it again, but it didn't work anymore. It was like I'd lost the momentum. I thought, 'Oh my God, what have I done?!' About a year later, I tried taking the medication again, but it didn't work. I guess I only had one chance. For a while, though, I thought malic acid and Zantac were a miracle."

Mari's worst symptom is the inability to handle noisy places and crowds. Simple activities that most people take for granted, such as going to the grocery story (with all its smells and colors) or even talking on the telephone while the television is on in the background, often send her into stimulation overload. Mari has only enough concentration to perform one task at a time. Trying to do two things at once makes her confused, especially if she has to talk on the phone and write a message at the same time. Fatigue only feeds the confusion.

Constant upset stomach and irritable bowel are the hardest parts of FM and CFS that Andrea has to bear. There's nothing worse than wanting to eat dinner but being so nauseated by the smell of the food on your plate that you want to vomit. Her diarrhea often comes on without warning. People who have survived a building fire often look for the exits whenever they enter a new place. Likewise, Andrea scans for the restroom wherever she can. The situation that most sets her tummy off is being stuck behind a big pick-up truck that's blowing exhaust fumes in her face. Andrea has had to pull off the road and wait for the offending vehicle to leave.

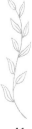

Such situations can trigger FM or CFS to flare up even when we've had our symptoms under control. For example, some people reported that they've put in a lot of hard work to enable themselves to make that hated trip to the grocery store. They go only when they feel well enough to do so. But standing in line behind a person who's wearing too much perfume can instantly cause their symptoms to flare. All that hard work on managing symptoms then goes out the window.

Nonetheless, minor adjustments have allowed many patients to better manage their symptoms. One person reported that she never returns phone calls until after she has had her afternoon nap. Another person said that he doesn't drive in rush-hour traffic. A third person confided that she will walk a block out of her way to avoid passing a person who is smoking a cigarette.

Little tricks like these allow you to get through your day with as few flare-ups as possible. Managing your symptoms requires eternal vigilance, however, and must often be done several times throughout the day. Try to anticipate situations that trigger your worst symptoms, and avoid them if at all possible. Your number-one priority is to prevent the aggravation of your pain and fatigue.

A Patient's Story: Lucy J.

Lucy J., who has FM, is forty-seven years old and has one son. She is training to be a hypnotherapist and lives in Bothell, Washington.

In 1973, I was hit by a semi truck, and that's when the pain began. It started during my early twenties, and it's been with me for the last twenty-seven years.

I began having headaches and pain in my neck, which I still have to this day. The doctors told me at the time that I had a whiplash injury that would clear up within a few months. However, one orthopedic surgeon did tell me that he didn't see any damage to my vertebrae and neck at the time of the original injury. He told me that

42

within five years they might be able to pick up some additional problems on X-rays, though.

I was diagnosed with FM about six years ago. I have not been diagnosed with CFS, and no doctors have even gone through its symptoms or talked to me about CFS. However, I have a tremendous amount of fatigue from the FM. I am fatigued all the time, depending on the quality of rest I get at night, which is usually pretty bad. I don't get good, quality sleep, so I usually wake up more exhausted than I was when I went to bed.

I used to have chronic daily headaches, but, luckily, I no longer do. I do have a chronic neck ache and upper backache on the right side of my body. Sometimes the pain is fairly mild, and other times it is intense. It depends on my level of activity that day. I cannot work part of the time because of the pain. I've had to quit numerous jobs because of it.

In the past, my doctors didn't connect my symptoms or realize that they came from the same syndrome. They just treated me on a symptom-by-symptom basis.

I take a lot of different medications (thirteen, on a regular basis). I have taken Prozac off and on for about twelve years, and it has helped my pain more than anything else. I also take an anti-inflammatory and an antiseizure medication, which is supposed to counteract my migraines, and it seems to be working well—I haven't had a migraine in weeks. I also take methadone for pain.

I'm extremely sensitive to smells and light. Sometimes I have to wear sunglasses; at one time I thought this was just related to my migraines (you tend to be more sensitive to light if you're susceptible to migraines). Certainly I'm very aware of pollution and any kind of particulate in the air, but previously I didn't know this was related to FM. I have very sensitive skin and sensitive tender points all over my body. But they usually don't bother me unless they're touched. I have a lot of stomach and intestinal problems, and irritable bowel syndrome, too. I go through bouts of diarrhea and constipation, but I pretty much stay on the diarrhea side of things.

I have a lot of foot problems; my feet hurt when I walk. I don't

43

know if that's related to the FM or if that's an early sign of arthritis. I have aches in my large joints, too. When I try to garden or do housework, I have a lot of lower-back pain (I can't do much gardening anymore). This pain doesn't constantly nag me, as the rest of the symptoms do, and it may be age-related. I also have a lot of memory problems. Sometimes I have good days. Right now it's pretty bad, though. The pain is just stabbing me.

I've pretty much suffered alone all of these years, thinking that the doctors couldn't find anything because I had some kind of neurosis. I've seen about fifteen doctors for this problem. They told me I had a chronic pain problem that I developed because of stress and nervous tension. FM is a very complex syndrome, but I feel that I was badly treated over the years, which wasn't due to negligence but to ignorance on the part of the medical profession.

Once I was properly diagnosed and I started to understand FM and educate myself, I realized that it has to be managed through a variety of techniques. I had to be persistent in finding a good doctor who knew how to help me manage my symptoms. One of the things that helped me most is the realization that it's not in my head, and that there are a lot of different ways to manage all the symptoms that I have.

Chapter 3

Conventional Therapies

WHILE THIS BOOK FOCUSES predominantly on alternative therapies, that should in no way discourage you from trying the full range of options available, including more traditional treatments such as pharmaceutical drugs. It's taken us a lot of time and effort to find the combination of conventional and unconventional treatments that works best. Many of the patients we interviewed for this book reported some level of relief from conventional remedies such as drugs and physical therapy, and it's worthwhile for everyone to give them a try as well.

For us, following the conventional wisdom on treating FM and CFS meant subjecting our bodies to many different kinds of drugs. There is no standard pharmaceutical treatment for all people with FM and CFS: what works for one person may only make another person worse. Trial and error is the only way to find a medication that may give some relief. As an illustration of the number of treatments that

45

you might try, we've included below a partial list of the drugs we've taken (the common use is in parentheses, and the use for FM/CFS follows):

- methadone (narcotic analgesic), for pain relief

- MS-Contin (pain medication)

- Oxycodone (narcotic analgesic), for pain relief

- Oxycontin (narcotic analgesic), for pain relief

- Procaine injections (anesthetic), for pain relief

- Ultram (opiate agonist), for pain relief

- Vicodin (narcotic analgesic), for pain relief

- Duragesic (a fentanyl patch used to distribute pain medication)

- cortisone injections (steroid), to reduce inflammation

- Prozac (antidepressant, used for pain relief and sleep)

- Serzone (antidepressant, used for pain relief and sleep)

- Trazodone (antidepressant, used for pain relief and sleep)

- Wellbutrin (antidepressant, used for pain relief and sleep)

- Zoloft (antidepressant, used for pain relief and fatigue)

- Naprosyn (anti-inflammatory, used for pain relief)

- Toradol (anti-inflammatory, used for pain relief)

- Flexeril (muscle relaxant)

- Norflex (muscle relaxant)

- Neurontin (treats seizures), for neurotransmitter regulation

- Sinemet (Parkinson's disease), for restless leg syndrome

- guaifenesin (expectorant), to remove wastes from muscles

- cholac lactulose syrup (treats constipation)

- Correctol ("the women's 'gentle' laxative")

- Kaopectate (treats diarrhea)

We've also kept the vitamin and supplement industry solvent for another fifty years by buying pills from A to Z:

- antioxidants (increase cell function by eliminating harmful free radicals)

- Chinese herbs (used to flush toxins from the body)

- evening primrose oil (an essential fatty acid that helps transport oxygen across membranes and acts as an anti-inflammatory)

- ginkgo biloba (enhances oxygen availability and aids in memory)

- magnesium (aids in muscle function)

- MSM (methyl sulfonyl methane used for muscle pain relief)

- Pro-Energy (a combination of magnesium and malic acid used for muscle pain relief)

- Super Blue Green Algae (for energy)

- vitamin B complex (for energy)

- vitamin C (supports the adrenal gland and immune system function)

- vitamin E (helps lubricate cells)

- zinc (supports immune system function)

We also tried these techniques:

- chiropractic adjustments

- heat and ice packs

- physical therapy

- psychotherapy

- surgery

Some of the drugs we tried had side effects that were worse than the symptoms we were trying to treat. But we were so desperate for relief that we willingly took these drugs and hoped for the best, despite the threat (in some cases) of liver toxicity, physical dependence, and unknown long-term side effects.

A majority of the drugs used to treat FM and CFS are prohibitively expensive for the person without medical insurance. Even patients with insurance report that they are frequently denied coverage of a particular medication for one reason or another. One of the most popular reasons is that the drug is "non-formulary," which means that it is entirely excluded from coverage. Most often, this simply means that the drug is expensive and the insurance company doesn't want to pay for it. Insurance companies especially balk at paying for narcotics, other medications prescribed on a long-term basis, or those prescribed "off-label" by the physician. (Almost any man in this country has the impotence drug Viagra covered by his insurance, but just try to get coverage for expensive narcotics to treat chronic pain!)

People whom we interviewed reported complex searches for the right medications and therapies. Melinda N., for example, who has FM, tried numerous pain medications before settling on methadone. She still takes it, along with others for sleep, headaches, and stomach problems. "I also take Trazodone; it helps my sleep disorder. It takes the edge off my pain, too. I tried Elavil [another antidepressant], but it made me gain weight. I get migraines, so I take Sumatriptan, 25 milligrams. For irritable bowel syndrome, I take 20 milligrams of Dicyclomine. I get this bloated gas feeling, which hurts my stomach; if I take a Dicyclomine, I might be able to cut the swelling down by about half. No matter what you take, you have to try the cheapest brand first with your HMO, and you have to go through a lot of extra grief to get what works."

Andrew M., a former electronics technician who also has FM, says that he and his doctor have been working on finding the right combination of medications. "I take two different kinds of antidepressants: one to treat my depression and one that's supposed to help with FM. I take Prozac for depression, and nortriptyline is the one I take for FM. Before bed, I also take two antihistamines. And I take 600 milligrams of guaifenesin twice a day, which is an experimental therapy that helps FM symptoms; it's supposed to work for 70 percent of patients. This is what I recommend the most. [Note: It is important for people to remember not to use any salicylates, such as aspirin products, while taking guaifenesin, as it counteracts the effects.]

Becky R. tried conventional drugs in conjunction with a naturopathic approach. "It was hard when my doctor first put me on Paxil, because I know it's an antidepressant," she says. "It was depressing to hear that I was depressed, and it took me a long time to come to terms with that. I thought, 'Okay, somebody labeled me depressed,' so I felt like I needed to sit down and cry, and I did. I was kind of worried that I would be stigmatized. The diagnosis of depression carries some baggage. Then one of my best friends came over and said, 'Look, take the medicine. You've got to get better. If it helps, then accept it.'"

Sherry J., who has both FM and CFS, says that she has no trouble relying on conventional medications to ease her pain. "I will honestly say that I live on Ultram. Before Ultram came along, my quality of life was about half of what it is now. I use it in two ways: as pain relief and as a stimulant. I now have a window of about five good hours a day, but the rest of my day is useless.

"I have always been very lucky; I've had a doctor almost from the beginning who believed me. But I had to go from one doctor to another until I found one who knew anything about this. All they allowed me for pain was one Tylenol 3 a day, for fifteen years. [Regarding opiate drugs,] I think it's a farce when they talk about addiction.

"When I started taking an antianxiety drug, a small amount every day, my migraines stopped altogether. My other medications are 150 milligrams of Zoloft, 7.5 milligrams of BuSpar twice a day, and one Tylenol 3 and two Ultrams when I get up in the morning. I use Chlorazopate, a very mild tranquilizer, at night to help myself sleep. In the last few months I've gone from one to two pills, because I've been on it for so many years it's not working as well. It's very important to me to get enough sleep. I have a urinary problem, so I have to make a lot of trips to the bathroom at night."

Sherry also takes vitamin and mineral supplements. "My supplements are Ultra C complex, Ultra B complex, and Ultra 2, a mixed mineral supplement that has everything in it," she says. "I buy everything through CFIDS & FM Health Resource [see Resources] because my money goes back into research and it's easier for me to get things in the mail. I also take calcium citrate, magnesium, malic acid, and CoQ10 [an antioxidant that supports cell function] every day. I tried DHEA [a hormone that helps increase energy and enhance the immune system], but I could not feel anything change. I also take ginkgo biloba, one or two a day. I've added that in the last few months because my cognitive problems are so bad. At times, when I have a flare-up with my hands, I use evening primrose oil capsules."

In contrast, some people we interviewed have not tried a variety of medications or explored a range of alternative therapies. For example, there's Dennis H., who has CFS. "I've been a support group leader for several years. It seems as if everybody in the group has tried something different, a change in diet, a specific medication, a dietary supplement. If somebody had luck with something, I would try it, but I haven't tried the more aggressive treatments. I haven't tried the 'alternatives,' either, like yoga, *tai chi*, or acupuncture. Other people are much more aggressive about trying all different kinds of treatments—some of which I am very uncomfortable with, like intramuscular injections or a lot of medications.

"In my support group, I view myself as the control subject; everyone else receives the experimental drugs and I am in the placebo group. I really am conservative; I never even liked to take aspirin or Tylenol or Excedrin on a regular basis. I consider myself lucky that I have a moderate case, even though it's severe enough that I can't work and my activities are cut back significantly."

Your search for the right combination of medication and therapies may be a difficult one, but, like the contributors to this book, you will find techniques that work. If your physician is only willing to try conventional therapies, take advantage of them, but remember to explore the many alternatives described elsewhere in this book as well. The combination of traditional and nontraditional therapies will work better than either will by itself.

Chapter 4

Osteopathy and Chiropractic Therapies

O STEOPATHY AND CHIROPRACTIC can be beneficial for anyone, especially people with FM and
CFS. Both therapies involve hands-on manipulation of the body, which helps you to achieve proper body
alignment, increases blood flow to injured areas, and can impart
a stronger sense of well-being. In this chapter, we hope to persuade you that these "alternative" treatments can work wonders when
done properly. For some people, relief is instantaneous; others must
be willing to continue treatment for months and sometimes years, if
necessary, before the full healing benefit can be attained.

Chiropractic is a health-care system that deals with the relationship between the spinal column and the nervous system. In order for
a person to experience harmony, vitality, and good health, there must
be an unobstructed flow of nerve impulses from the brain through the
spinal nerves and out to every part of the body. Misalignments (sub-

luxations) cause interference in the transmission of nerve impulses from the brain to the organs and other body tissues. When nerve transmission to a particular organ or part of the body is interrupted for long periods of time, it causes impaired bodily function and results in pain and illness. Chiropractic can help by addressing underlying spinal problems. It is the largest drugless nonsurgical health-care system in the Western world.

Osteopathy is a system of medicine based on the theory that disturbances in the musculoskeletal system affect other body parts and can cause many disorders. These disturbances can be corrected by various hands-on manipulative techniques, used in conjunction with conventional therapeutic procedures such as medication and physical therapy. A doctor of osteopathy specializes in, among other things, the use of osteopathic manipulation. An osteopath treats a patient by moving various body parts in a normal range of motion. The doctor also places his or her hands on the patient's scalp, using a gentle "rocking" motion to manipulate the cranial bones. This stimulates tiny muscles and nerve endings in the scalp to help effect proper cranial alignment.

We and the people interviewed for this book have had very positive experiences with both techniques. Mari, for example, has had years of chiropractic care. "When I was eighteen years old, I had terrible sciatica," Mari said. After suffering with it for weeks, she went to a chiropractor. "After a few visits, the pain was gone, and I was a believer," she says. "Since then, I've made chiropractic a big part of my overall treatment plan. I go twice a week for adjustments, and that helps alleviate my headaches and helps me stay flexible. I have an ongoing problem with a rib that pops out of place. Between chiropractic adjustment and exercise, I've been able to keep the pain at a dull roar rather than at a debilitating level. My chiropractors have shown me strengthening exercises to complement my treatment. It's been my experience that these help to 'hold' the adjustment in place and keep tight muscles from pulling the vertebrae out of alignment.

"If I miss a visit or two, I have a lot more body stiffness," Mari says. "I get a lot more headaches. I had a lot of foot pain, which I think arose from my back pain, but with regular chiropractic visits,

53

the foot pain has calmed down. People with FM have stiff and tense muscles, which causes their joints to not work properly. Chiropractic adjustment can help this problem.

"When you're looking for a chiropractor, make sure they know how to treat FM and CFS. Ask the chiropractor if he or she has any FM or CFS patients, and what specific treatment plan they recommend.

"I definitely recommend chiropractic as part of anyone's treatment plan," Mari says. "People shouldn't be afraid of the adjustment process; you may instantly feel better, and it never hurts. Also, a lot of insurance plans have to cover chiropractic visits now."

Andrea has had a positive experience with osteopathy. "Four months after being rear-ended in a car accident, I was having tremendous pain in my head, neck, shoulders, and upper back," Andrea says. "I had to beg my primary care physician just to get an X-ray done. The technician took one look at the X-ray and said, 'You know, I'm not qualified to interpret these, but something just doesn't look right to me.' She looked in her book and pointed to an X-ray of a normal cervical vertebrae. Then she pointed to my X-ray and showed me that the vertebrae in my neck were literally pulled almost a half-inch apart.

"Since I had been working with a massage therapist at the time, I told her about the misalignment," Andrea says. "She recommended that I see an osteopathic physician to help get my vertebrae back in line. Had I known at the time that I would be going weekly for almost two years (at $190 an hour), I probably would never have gone at all. But I did go, religiously, and I believe it made all the difference in the world. I would arrive at the osteopath's office with a headache, dizziness, muscle pain and spasms, leg pain, foot pain—you name it, I had a pain in it. She used gentle manipulation, and slowly, gradually, week after week, month after month, year after year, the muscles relaxed a little, and the vertebrae were slowly realigned." Andrea's situation was acute, and it took her a long time to achieve her treatment goals. You may not have to make this time commitment, depending upon your situation.

Erin P., who has FM, says that she got more relief from chiropractic because she used it in conjunction with other therapies. "Most of the pain in my body is gone, although that was also relieved early on by some other things," she says. "Chiropractic helped me a lot over a long period of time, but I think I had more relief in a shorter period of time by going to a physical therapist who practiced Feldenkrais. That's a movement therapy. I went in because of my knees and came out with almost a whole new body. It was amazing."

Melinda N., who also has FM, sees a chiropractor to help keep her limber and able to exercise. "I was very surprised, because I didn't think he would help me, but he has," Melinda says. "I had real frustration with my hip for two and a half years, because my hip was rotated and healed improperly after the [car] accident. But my current chiropractor seems to have unlocked that area. I'm freed up and I can do belly-dancing moves with a lot less pain and execute them better."

Treatment for FM and CFS takes time. It takes diligence. It takes patience. It takes an overwhelming desire to be well. It also takes money and referrals and insurance and reimbursements. Both of us were fortunate enough to find treatment providers who were incredibly skilled and dedicated. Osteopathy and chiropractic care have given us functionality and relief from pain that we probably wouldn't have had otherwise.

Chiropractic Technique

Dr. Robert Freitas

Dr. Robert Freitas is a chiropractor and owner of the Sea View Chiropractic Clinic in West Seattle. He received his certification in Spinal Industrial Disability Evaluation at the Los Angeles College of Chiropractic in 1987.

Chiropractic students graduate with around 400 hours of training in radiology, compared to a general practitioner medical doctor, who has about sixty to eighty hours. We also learn to do a lot of hands-on motion palpation. Basically, we learn what a normal spine and normal joints feel like, and what the muscles that move those joints feel like. We look for what we call "subluxations." Actually, a subluxation can also be called joint dysfunction, joint adhesion, or joint fixation.

Before we treat a patient, we take a patient history, a past and present medical history, and a family history; then there is a standard orthopedic neurological screening for any pathological problems. Then there is the chiropractic portion, which is motion palpation—that's when we run joints through a normal range of motion and feel how they move or don't move. We feel for trigger points, what we call "hot spots," in muscles and tendons. If it is warranted and if pathological signs are there, we may also do X-rays. X-rays don't tell me what isn't moving, but they show me pathology and reasons to adjust or not adjust the spine.

Basically, there are three kinds of joint motion: active (when you can move your own joint), passive (when the practitioner takes the joint into his or her own hands to see how it moves), and physiological (when the chiropractor manipulates the joint to reduce or improve motion). In other words, I take people to their active range of motion, and then I passively bring the joint to the point where it's fixated, where it does not move any further, and then I make the adjustment, a quick, forceful thrust into that physiological plane, thus restoring normal joint motion. It's a very short thrust, just a fraction of an inch, and as it's done we hear an audible pop.

Current theory holds that there is nitrogen inside the joint, compressed into a liquid state. When we adjust the joint, or what we call "gap the joint," the pop that we hear is actually gases expanding inside the joint, allowing it to move freely again. We are also breaking up minor adhesions in the ligaments around the joint and joint capsule.

I believe chiropractic adjustments can help people with FM and CFS. I don't think it can cure the problems, but we can offer some relief. In people with FM, the joint is not out of place; it is literally stuck in its normal range of motion. That causes aberrant motion or changes the axis of motion in the joint, which in turn causes abnormal motion and puts stresses on the joint capsule, ligaments and muscles that move the joint.

During treatment, the patient usually lies face down, since we're working on the spine; however, there are many different positions. The body has to be put in different positions to address the joint play, and one joint can have several planes of motion. Which way we turn or position a person depends on the plane of motion in which the joint is fixed.

When people react to pain, they get tense, and their muscles go into contracture, causing joints to move abnormally. And as a joint moves abnormally, it puts even more stress on itself, which causes more reactive muscle spasm, or splinting. A vicious cycle has just started. The joint adjustment we do reduces tightness by improving joint function and allowing the muscles and tendons that move the joint to relax. In my practice, I also use moist heat and muscle stretching, along with some deep-tissue work, to improve joint mobilization. Through this work, I'm stimulating neurons called mechanoreceptors, and a feedback loop is established that reduces or relaxes muscles and tissues around the joint.

The only time chiropractic hurts is when you're in an acute, inflammatory state; when an injury has just happened, for example. But even in an acute situation, it is important to maintain motion. A good example of this is surgery. The doctor sutures you up, and when you're walking around the next day, you feel like you're pulling your stitches out. That hurts, but you're putting normal stress on the body that enables it to heal along the lines of that stress. This is why we would adjust a patient who's in an acute state. It does hurt, but then again the patient is already hurting.

Sometimes chiropractic care is not appropriate. Chiropractors are well versed in determining the stability of a sprain, grading the sprain I, II, III, or IV. If a joint is totally unstable and they can't even lift it against gravity, of course it needs to be supported by a splint. And if there's gross inflammation and bruising, chiropractors know that there are broken blood vessels and that the patient needs medication and medical care. In a grade I or grade II sprain, however, there is generally no disruption of the tendons, and chiropractic manipulation is indicated.

Chiropractic care is recommended before the body has time to react to an injury; an injury can become a chronic problem, because the muscles have memory. I believe that this is one of the components of FM and CFS: the body develops a kind of "pain memory" that lowers the stress threshold. Whether this memory is a nerve memory or a chemical change doesn't matter; a lot of people develop FM after an injury, so their bodies are reacting to the trauma. They have a type of "allergic reaction" to the body's own inflammatory process, and a kind of chronic state or memory develops. In order to prevent this, any type of joint mobilization is beneficial in the first stages after an injury.

Irritability in the muscles causes joint fixation and creates a cycle of pain. When you get a joint adjusted, you will feel better. We know that adjustment of the spine actually sends inhibitory responses that relax the muscles for up to seventy-two hours after an adjustment. Researchers have proven this with skin galvanic sensing units, the kind used in biofeedback.

Everybody is different, of course, and benefits depend on what part of the body has been injured. If, for instance, a joint fixation has not allowed proper motion at a segment that has parasympathetic nerves associated with it, you will get dramatic relief after an adjustment. But if that association isn't there, the adjustment may help, you may feel a little better, but you won't get that overall feeling of well-being.

In most instances, people with FM and CFS should at least try chiropractic, because if their muscles are hyperirritable, tense, and fibrotic, their joints will not move as they should. This causes biomechanical disturbances. Chiropractic won't cure the problem, but patients benefit from more restful sleep patterns and an increased feeling of relaxation.

Some techniques are more beneficial than others for people with FM or CFS. For example, gentle osseous mobilization is better than forcible techniques for the patient who is already in significant pain. The activator, a tool that chiropractors use to adjust the spine, is probably not going to change the biomechanics right away, so we probably wouldn't use it on people with those kinds of problems.

Find a chiropractor with specific experience in dealing with CFS or FM. If they have dealt with these syndromes before, and if they do some soft-tissue work (in which they feel where the tender points are), then they are probably well versed in such treatment.

Getting Relief with Osteopathy

Dr. Cathy Lindsay

Dr. Cathy Lindsay is a licensed osteopathic physician in private practice in Seattle. During her ten-year practice, she has helped hundreds of patients to return to functionality and a greater level of health.

Osteopathy differs from chiropractic manipulation. Chiropractors tend to believe that everything originates at the spine and is related to spinal alignment or irritation of the spinal nerves. The focus of chiropractic is bringing the spinal column back into alignment; the focus is on bony adjustment. (This varies, depending on the individual chiropractor and his or her specific focus.) Osteopathic treatment finds restrictions and things that are out of alignment anywhere in the body, and then does body work to help realign them. It works on a structural level, but it also works because the body is a whole organism—everything is interrelated, and the body has an inherent healing mechanism that works best when all parts of the body are moving freely.

Thorough diagnostic evaluation is completed before any osteopathic treatment is started. We begin with a full medical history, an injury history, and a birth history. We also do a thorough assessment of the patient's current symptoms (why they came to see the osteopath), and we do a review of body systems just to see what other things are going on. Then we do what's called an "osteopathic structural evaluation," as well as a brief neurological evaluation. These evaluations assess the relationship between structure and function in the body. We look for areas of misalignment as well as functional restriction and freedom of motion—we look at how your body actually moves when it's taken through its full range of motion. Then, using those structural and functional assessments, we treat the relationship

59

between the body's soft and bony tissues. If we find things that are worth addressing with osteopathic treatment, we begin treatment on the first visit.

Treatment is hard to describe until you've actually experienced it for yourself. Usually it's pretty gentle; I use a fairly subtle approach. Many of the treatments are simply gentle movements of the body, and we actually use the body as a director that tells us where to move the patient in order to free up restrictions or unwind twists in the connective tissue, and to get things back in alignment. For some people, treatment is so gentle that they think I haven't done anything. But they leave and think, "Wow, I guess she did," because they're sore, feel better, or notice some change.

Osteopathy is different than some other body-work methods that try to directly break up restrictions in the body. In part, it's a more effective therapy than some other approaches *because* it is so gentle. We do have some direct approaches, and spinal manipulation is one of them. (I don't tend to use it as much because I don't need it.) Osteopathy doesn't tend to irritate the tissues as much as other therapies, though, and in people with FM the tissues tend to be easily irritated. However, there is no specific approach for any condition, including FM. All patients are treated as unique individuals. Sometimes osteopathy helps people with conditions such as FM and CFS, and sometimes it doesn't. It depends on the individual and what trauma may have contributed to their condition.

Trauma can adversely impact the body's function, which can in turn affect a person's health. Trauma can create low-back problems, breathing and digestive disorders, headaches, or menstrual problems. Treating the body with osteopathic manipulation after a trauma can help return movement to the bones in the head and pelvis, which will then allow the body to return to its pretrauma state of function.

The craniosacral approach, which uses hands-on manipulation, was developed by osteopaths. This therapy focuses on the cranium and its relationship to the rest of the body, and works with the bones and membrane attachments in the head. After a hands-on manipulation of this kind, the patient's own healing processes may actually become more effective, and we can effect a general sense of well-being and overall health in the patient.

When I perform an osteopathic treatment, I apply gentle pressure to the tailbone or head of the patient to try and unblock any restrictions I may find. I can also use this type of treatment on any area of the body, not just the cranium or the tailbone.

The relationship between the bones of the skull and how it affects the body's overall health was discovered in the late 1930s by an osteopath, Will Sutherland, who was a student of Andrew Taylor Still, who founded osteopathic medicine in the 1800s. John Upledger, another osteopath, developed his own approach to the cranial method and subsequently founded the Upledger Institute in Florida. He coined the term "craniosacral therapy" and was the first person to train non-physicians to perform craniosacral work. Craniosacral therapists who aren't physicians usually receive their training at the Upledger Institute. Thus people who do other kinds of bodywork are now being trained in this approach, as well as physicians, who may be trained with more of a diagnostic focus.

▪ A Patient's Story: Barbara M.

Barbara is thirty-seven years old and has FM and CFS. She works part-time as an antiques dealer and lives in Issaquah, Washington. Chiropractic has helped her manage her pain.

I first heard about CFS years ago, when they were calling it "yuppie flu." I started to notice all these symptoms.

I had terrible bouts of insomnia, even though I was exhausted, because my legs jumped around so much. I've always had restless-leg syndrome; I had it by the time I was ten. It's increased over the years until my legs actually ache and hurt, and the pain has gone up into my arms and shoulder blades. I've had headaches and migraines my whole life, complicated by the fact that I've had a lot of head injuries. I've been treated for irritable bowel syndrome since I was a teenager,

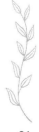

although lately I've had that pretty much under control. I'm more careful about what I eat and how I eat; I know which foods I have to avoid.

But until I was diagnosed with both FM and CFS, I never knew that all of these symptoms were part of the same problem. Before the diagnosis, I'd begun doing a lot of research on my own, and I started to see the words "CFS" and "Epstein-Barr virus." But most of the books that I read were about how to cope with it, not how to cure it. What I really wanted was someone to give me a diet and exercise plan, some ideas for medications, or something I could actively do to change the CFS; I didn't want somebody to hold my hand and commiserate with me.

I became very disgusted with the medical profession, especially since they missed the fact that I had had a severely broken tailbone since I was about fourteen years old. It had never been straightened, never been diagnosed. The bottom couple of inches were smashed for years. I had sciatica when I was in college. I had a terrible time sitting in lectures, and I was sent to gynecologists because the sciatica was pinching nerves and pulling muscles. I was complaining about terrible pain around my lower back on both sides and into the front of my groin. They even did a colonoscopy. I also had a laparoscopy, where they go in through the navel and check the ovaries. But despite all of the doctors I saw and all the exams I had, nobody even mentioned the broken tailbone.

After learning that doctors don't know all that you think they know, and they're not as informed on things as you expect them to be, I was pretty disillusioned with the medical system. So I tried to learn more from books, hoping that somebody would have breakthrough knowledge that the doctors didn't have. At that time, I didn't know of a doctor who specialized in CFS, and each time I saw a new general practitioner and asked about it, the doctor wasn't really receptive and didn't have any suggestions on it. Usually, they said that nobody's really sure if the Epstein-Barr virus causes CFS or if it's connected to mononucleosis. I heard a lot about that theory. There was also a lot of stigma attached to CFS at that time; it was sort of for whiners, and I didn't want to get lumped in with all those people.

I was diagnosed with rheumatoid arthritis when I was about twenty-one (although I think that was really FM). The doctor who diagnosed me put me on medication for a full year. He never even noticed the broken tailbone—even though it stuck out in a big lump. The only thing the medicine did was permanently stain my teeth. Finally, I just threw the medicine away, and a friend took me to a chiropractor.

As soon as I walked in, he said he could tell I had a broken tailbone by the way I had built up a mass on top of my shoulders and by the way that I stood. He told me that I had the most severely broken tailbone he'd ever seen. He straightened it, and for the first time I wasn't in complete agony. He couldn't believe that nobody had ever diagnosed it, especially when I'd been complaining for six or seven years about lower-back pain and sciatica.

I was always sent to individual specialists, but no one ever said, "Hey, there's a connection between all these things." I always felt self-conscious when I went to a doctor and had to explain what was wrong, like I was a hypochondriac or something. I knew something was wrong, but I wondered, "Is it just me, or do other people have the same thing? Or do I have a whole bunch of problems that the 'normal' person doesn't have?" I've just kind of kept my mouth shut because I feel like I'm not getting anywhere anyway. Plus, if you tell too many doctors too many complaints, they don't believe any of them.

I have a nice friend who is in the same leaky boat, and in the past several years I've met other people who have similar problems; they're not just whiners and they don't have the "disease of the month" or anything like that. We're not crazy, and I know we have something that medicine hasn't really caught up with yet.

But being sick has made me really appreciate the times when I'm feeling good. I appreciate it when people around me are happy, too. Life has definitely taught me to make the most of those times. It's given me more patience with other people. I've gone through phases of being mad at God because I have this problem I can't fix, even though I've tried really hard. But then I remember that there are people who have terminal cancer or are paralyzed. I try to not get bogged down in self-pity, because it doesn't help. Besides, everybody has some-

63

thing wrong with them. I try to do what's intelligent and what's helpful in coping with my problems and alleviating them as best I can.

For people like us, inertia is one of the biggest enemies. It makes you give in to your negative feelings, and you wallow in the pain and misery. It makes you disappointed when plans go awry or you have to give them up. And if you think about all the limitations that are upon you, rather than the opportunities, you can actually intensify the pain and inertia that you're feeling. When I go through a really long phase of feeling unwell, I have to crawl out of a deep rut, come back into the light, and start living again.

Chapter 5

Chinese Medicine

I N THIS CHAPTER, we explain the various remedies available under the Chinese treatment philosophy. Traditional Chinese medicine is a system of treatment, thought, and practice that has existed for thousands of years. Its disciplines include acupuncture, herbal therapy, nutrition, massage, and movement therapies such as *tai chi* and *chi kung*. These individual therapies all share a philosophy that the body is an interconnected organism and should be treated holistically, rather than on the symptom-by-symptom basis that Western medicine tends to use.

The Chinese believe that the body contains energy, a life force called *chi. Chi* can become imbalanced, stuck, or deficient in a number of ways. When this happens, physical conditions that we refer to as illness can develop. There are five major categories of *chi*: organ *chi*, which is the *chi* that energizes each of our organs; acupuncture meridian *chi*, which is energy that circulates throughout the meridian pathways of the body; nutritive *chi*, which you get from food; protective *chi*, also known as "superficial" *chi*, which defends the body from illness, regulates body temperature, and protects the body from germs in the environment; and ancestral *chi*, which is the *chi* you are born with that is given to you by your parents.

People all over the world turn to Chinese medicine when they are sick, but Mari's first experience with it left a little to be desired. She decided to try it because the more conventional therapies had failed to ease the pain in her feet, and she felt that she had nothing to lose. On the advice of a friend, Mari headed to a healer in Chinatown. "A friend told me about a traditional Chinese healer, an elderly man with amazing healing energy. My friend trusted him completely," Mari says. "The place looked like an old garage, with huge storage containers of brown, dried things sitting all over. The healer told me, 'Buy fresh chicken feet, boil them with garlic, and drink the juice.'"

"'Chicken feet for your feet,' he kept saying, smiling all the time." Mari says she was so desperate that she actually tried it—six times! She reports, not surprisingly, that this was like drinking a big glass of hot, dirt-flavored chicken fat. She also experienced no change in the pain in her feet. However, the Chinese doctor gave her a helpful *chi kung* exercise that she does to this day.

Mari also tried acupuncture to treat her pain. "I was unable to continue very long with the treatments, because my acupuncturist moved," she says. "But I quickly got relief for my digestive problems. It was my first experience with moxa [an herb that is burned to add heat to the body] and the cupping technique [used to draw blood to the surface]. I experienced a feeling of peace and relaxation while I was getting the acupuncture treatments. In some sites, I would experience a 'rush' of energy, but never pain. I got relief for my depression, too, with the use of ear points. These are tiny metal studs that are inserted into an acupuncture point in the ear and left for several days."

The Chinese have successfully used herbs to treat illness for thousands of years. Ellen J. said she takes numerous herbs every day to help combat her symptoms of FM and CFS. The herbs Ellen has taken include the following:

- astragalus *(huang chi)*, to increase energy and build resistance to disease

- *dong quai*, for treatment of ovarian cysts, menstrual cramps, and insomnia

- licorice *(gan t'sao)*, for treatment of stomach problems and adrenal exhaustion; helps to heal liver damage from illness and poisons

- ginger root, for digestion

- turmeric, an anti-inflammatory that helps with digestion

- linden flowers, which strengthen the lungs

Chinese medicine, especially acupuncture, has tremendous potential to alleviate pain and stiffness. Andrea reports positive experiences with Chinese medicine and acupuncture; in fact, she trusts them more than Western methods. Andrea remembers that she would go in for a treatment that involved getting needles stuck all over her body, but she would immediately fall asleep. She would wake up feeling refreshed and pain-free, even if only for a few days.

Many other Chinese therapies are now widely available. *Chi kung*, for example, was the first exercise form created in China, invented between three thousand and five thousand years ago, according to practitioner Kim Ivy. "It was created by people who observed how their bodies interacted with nature: when they got sick, when they felt good, what type of movements and breathing they could do that would better harmonize their bodies with the cycle of nature," Kim says. "So movement, meditation, and mindful breathing emerged, and their creators found that these things actually helped to strengthen their bodies. Concepts like the immune system were not necessarily thought about at the time, but *chi kung* came out of this very observant, meditative, slow-movement type of activity.

"Martial artists then began to study traditional Chinese medicine," Kim says. "Out of the *chi kung* and movement systems came the idea of acupuncture meridians and the Chinese way of looking internally at the body, at the meridians and internal organs. And so the martial artists became *chi kung* practitioners and doctors, and from that developed a martial art form that we know today as *tai chi*. There are a lot of different systems and styles, but basically *tai chi*, like *chi kung*, is a very slow-moving, harmonizing practice, in which the practitioner tries to harmonize his or her energy with the energy of a 'shadow partner.'"

Ann A., who has FM, says acupuncture helps relieve her pain. "In Chinese medicine, you're trying to correct the imbalances that cause pain, rather than just treating individual symptoms," she says. "I've noticed that over time it's really helped in terms of strengthening. I feel like I'm stronger at the core. My acupuncturist's treatments can just zap pain right away. I'm also using some Chinese herbs. I have used two formulations [tinctures] that are a combination of traditional Chinese medicine and homeopathy. One of them supports the pineal gland, which is important for hormonal balance, and the gland that secretes melatonin. The second helps support those systems in the body that cope with external stressors."

Many people with FM and CFS have felt compelled to try Eastern medicine because Western medicine has largely failed us. We are so eager for help that we may try anything if it promises relief. While Chinese medicine hasn't proven to be a magic pill, we urge anyone with a chronic pain or fatigue syndrome to try acupuncture, *tai chi*, and maybe even *chi kung*. Many insurance companies now provide some reimbursement for acupuncture and other "alternative" treatments. This chapter is full of suggestions and affirmations designed to persuade the reader to give Chinese medicine a try.

Acupuncture

Sara Wicklein

Sara Wicklein is a licensed acupuncturist in private practice in Seattle.

Sara was an accountant working in corporate America when she became ill with hypoglycemia. She quit her high-stress job, graduated from acupuncture school at Bastyr University in 1993, and has been practicing ever since. She believes that Chinese medicine is all about balance, and that acupuncture works to get the body's energy back into a balanced range.

Acupuncture is the oldest nondrug health-care system in the world. This healing philosophy, which has been practiced for thousands of years, acknowledges the healing potential of the human body. When I became ill, a friend of mine was using acupuncture, so I thought I'd try it. It really did help me. I felt so much better that I became fascinated with acupuncture and how it worked.

Treatment involves the insertion of microthin needles into corresponding points on the body. From a Western-medicine perspective, there's no explanation for exactly how it works, but we do know that the energy in the body does shift when needles are used at specific acupuncture points. We can also get a similar effect from acupressure, which uses gentle pressure instead of needles at specific points on the body. But acupuncture is a little stronger, and for some conditions it is less painful than acupressure, because some areas are very tight and can be painful if we put pressure on them.

Sometimes people feel the actual needle when it goes in. Sometimes they don't. Some people feel a rush of energy, or heat, and sometimes they feel an electrical sensation. Some people feel hardly anything at all. Some people fall sound asleep within an instant of having the needle inserted; I've had patients I can hardly wake up after half an hour.

Acupuncture uses different types of needles; I use Japanese needles, which are a bit smaller than the others. Chinese needles are a bit sturdier. Some needles are bigger and longer than others, and so are the bodies that I use them on. Bigger needles are used, for example, on a person's hip, because the points are deeper there. If someone has sciatic pain, we need to get in there. But you don't really feel pain after the needle is in. I use heat-sterilized disposable needles—

they're used only once. Most acupuncturists use disposable needles, although some use the kind that are resterilized.

Adding heat during the session can help arthritis and muscle problems. The acupuncturist can also use a technique called "cupping," which uses small glass jars and heat to draw more blood into a particular area. We use two kinds of cups—one has a little pump out of which air is pulled, and the other is a cup-shaped glass object. We heat the air inside the cup with a flame, burning out the oxygen and making a vacuum, and put the cup over the area. This raises the skin under the cup and brings more blood into the area. This is especially helpful for muscle tension in the back and problems with lung congestion; it helps to bring things to the surface.

Some people feel pain relief almost immediately. With others, it takes more time. They might have four or five good days after treatment, and then they go downhill, but not to exactly where they were before.

There are more than four hundred specific places on the body that correspond to specific physical problems. Also, there are what we call "Ashii points." "Ashii" literally means "where it hurts." If someone twists an ankle, we use needles in corresponding places, but if there's a specific spot that hurts that's not a true acupuncture site, we'll still treat the injury. It helps to open up the energy around the injured area, so it can heal more quickly.

Because we do a long intake interview, the first acupuncture treatment usually lasts between an hour and fifteen minutes to an hour and a half. Return visits usually last between forty-five minutes and an hour; it depends on the person and how much discussion needs to take place. The actual treatment on the table takes about twenty minutes.

Acupuncture is just one part of Chinese medicine, which looks at the emotions and how they affect the body. Practitioners also look at external forces, such as the weather. We look at external pathogenic factors (viruses, bacteria, etc.). We look at the foods that you eat and how you eat: whether you sit down and take time to eat or just stuff food in your face and go.

There are also all kinds of Chinese herbs for all kinds of conditions: digestion, colds, flus, injured muscles. You name it, there's an herb for it. There's no single treatment that is perfect for everyone, though. We all have the power to heal inside ourselves; the mystery is what key will unlock it for each of us.

I think it's a good idea for people with FM and CFS to try acupuncture, but you really need to try at least two or three months of weekly treatments just to see what kind of relief you can get. To go for a shorter period of time won't be enough in this situation, because the body is out of balance, and it will take time for the body to process the new information that acupuncture will bring to it. It's also important to try all kinds of therapies and practitioners at the same time, like chiropractic, massage therapy, maybe even a spiritual advisor.

Visiting an acupuncturist is not as simple as just coming in and saying you have pain or digestive problems. I want to know if you have those symptoms, but I also want to know about all kinds of other things, like your sleep pattern, your emotional state before the illness, what went on in your life before this, what your childhood was like. Acupuncturists want to know all the pieces of the person. We don't look at just one thing, because Chinese medicine looks at the whole body.

A Patient's Story: Ellen J.

Ellen is a thirty-eight-year-old jewelry artist with a lifelong interest in natural/alternative health. Part magpie, she currently lives in Seattle, where she is surrounded by mountains, flowering plants, multicolored beads, and her pet rabbit, all of which help her to heal body and soul. She has FM and CFS.

After I seriously injured my lower back in 1992, I started going for acupuncture treatments twice a week. I thought the pain from muscle spasms would drive me out of my mind. The acupuncture treatments were the only thing that even began to help me cope with the tremendous pain caused by the injury, and the emotional distress I was experiencing because I was bedridden for months on end. Physical therapy aggravated my condition, and so I did this acupuncture therapy on the advice of the physician who was treating me for the back injury. I can now do both treatments in conjunction with each other.

I have gone for regular acupuncture treatments once a week for the past four years. I have been treated by acupuncturists from two different traditions: Chinese and Japanese. The difference is in the type of needle they use and how deeply the needling is done. Both have been very effective treatments for decreasing pain, getting over acute illnesses like sinus infections and the flu, helping me to cope with depression and express my anger, and improving my digestion. I notice that whenever I take a break from this treatment, I have less stamina and get infections much more often.

I take Chinese herbs and use principles of Chinese nutrition in my daily cooking. My acupuncturist has given me lists of foods that help to build and nourish *chi* and blood. Before trying Chinese nutrition, I was primarily a vegetarian. I now add a portion of fish or chicken to my meals once a week. I also eat many more root vegetables (sweet potato and parsnips) and work on balancing different flavors (sour, bitter, sweet, pungent, and salty). I make sure that the whole foods I eat are prepared in a way that best supports my particular needs. I use a lot of ginger, turmeric, and coriander in my cooking of squash, bean dishes, and soups to aid in digestion, and decrease pain and swelling in my joints and connective tissues. I eat steamed vegetables and brown rice when I need to detoxify from exposure to allergens and chemical toxins. I try to focus on using food to heal my body, rather than just eating on the run as fuel between activities, like I did before I got sick.

I also do Chinese stretching exercises, including *chi kung*. For a while, I did *tai chi*, but my budget only supports a certain number of treatments at a time, and I have trouble remembering the exercises well enough to do them at home alone.

I have also used homeopathic treatment as part of my medicinal arsenal for more than fifteen years. I started by reading books and trying various remedies. I regularly use the remedy *Arnica montana* for sore muscles and to prevent bruising after I bump into things. Before and after dental treatment and any surgical procedure, I use *Hypericium perfoliatum* to prevent and treat nerve pain and injury. I have used *Rhus toxicodendron* to relieve joint pain related to arthritis. I highly recommend a good basic book on homeopathy for anyone's home first-aid kit.

I have also been treated by homeopathic physicians and naturopathic physicians trained in homeopathy. They were interested in everything, from my thirst patterns to my dreams to the nature of my pain to my emotional responses and personal relationship patterns. They also took a very detailed history of all illnesses and symptoms that I had had throughout my life. After they had analyzed my symptoms to find the most appropriate remedy for my constitution, I was given a remedy that helped to heal the patterns of disease that my body/mind had developed. I was also warned that sometimes the remedies would provoke a sort of healing crisis in which I would reexperience the symptoms of my illnesses, only for a shorter period of time and in the reverse order that I had originally gotten them. I was told to expect that healing would take thirty to sixty days for each year that I had been alive. At the age of thirty-three, it would take up to sixty-six months before my body would reverse the disease pattern and be restored to health.

I have had some intense healing crises. Sometimes my pain was excruciating for a few days, but afterward I didn't have that particular type of pain again. I have reexperienced childhood allergy symptoms without being exposed to the original allergen, and then they have resolved. After each healing crisis, I have come through stronger and a little healthier. It was helpful to know what these episodes were; otherwise, I might have thought I was getting worse, or I might have taken lots of medicines to suppress the symptoms, making it that much harder for my body to heal its vital force. Sometimes, though, the remedies stopped working, and I had to be reevaluated to see if I needed to take the original remedy again or if I had moved on to a different remedy pattern.

▓ *Tai Chi* and *Chi Kung*

Kim Ivy

Kim Ivy is a certified *tai chi* and *chi kung* instructor and owns the Embrace the Moon school in Seattle.

Tai chi consists of physical exercises based on principles of rhythmic movement, equilibrium of body weight, and effortless breathing designed to build *chi* (vital life energy). Originally developed as a martial art for self-defense, it is characterized by moving slowly and continuously without strain through a sequence of contrasting movements. Each movement develops from the last and flows into the oncoming movement. The objective of *tai chi* is to achieve health and tranquillity through movement while developing the mind and body. It teaches the individual how to control the nervous system in order to put the entire body at rest. *Chi kung*'s specific exercises are designed to build *chi* and restore health.

Tai chi and *chi kung* help the body to relax from muscle spasm and injury. I've worked with hundreds of people who have had success with them. But neither works for everybody. *Tai chi* is a continuous-movement type of exercise, but you can stand in one place while doing *chi kung*. For people who have severe FM, *tai chi* is a bit better, because standing in one place and holding a posture is not good for them. For people who have chronic fatigue, *chi kung* tends to be a bit better, because less movement is involved.

When I moved to Seattle four years ago, a physician contracted me to develop a program using *tai chi* and *chi kung* for his chronic-pain patients. We wanted these people to have some sort of movement and exercise system that would give them pain relief and enable them to function without always having to come back to the pain clinic. Although we didn't expect it, most of the people who joined this program had CFS and FM. I worked with them extensively for six months to a year, and we learned how to integrate *tai chi* and *chi kung* for these types of chronic pain and fatigue syndromes.

74

We discovered that these treatments are good for people with FM and CFS because of the slowness of the exercises, which take the body very, very gently through a whole range of motions without engaging a strong muscle contraction, like weightlifting does. These types of exercises do not create adrenaline in the body. People who have FM know that if they engage in physical activities that produce adrenaline, their bodies have a difficult time processing that extra adrenaline. The slowness and "flowing" nature of *tai chi* and *chi kung* allow people to adjust and modify this type of exercise for their own body. For example, if your neck and shoulder area are in spasm, you would not want to raise your hands over your shoulders. *Tai chi* and *chi kung* actually work because the body learns to relax. And as the whole muscular system learns to relax, the internal organs are revitalized. The body can actually get exercise and still be in a state of relaxation.

Through the years, we have found these exercises to be most beneficial for people who have a variety of pain problems. When some people began at the school, they could hardly move. At first they would simply work on their breathing or on visualizing the movements. They would do a little bit of movement and then sit down. This type of activity is very noncompetitive; it doesn't have any kind of goal. People I work with who have taken the classes for several years have had incredible progress and have been able to engage in classes that are an hour long. They come three or four times a week, and, very slowly, their bodies are starting to open up to a full range of motion and are becoming energized.

Tai chi and *chi kung* are now extremely popular for people of all ages and fitness levels, but students really need to get a teacher with whom they can communicate, who understands their needs, who is willing to work with them to adapt the form to their needs. You can do these exercises many, many different ways, as long as you have a teacher who is willing to be flexible. If people have FM or CFS, I really don't recommend that they buy a videotape and try to learn that way. That's a good way of putting yourself into spasm, because it's very difficult to make your own posture and form correct.

I have observed that many of the FM points, or "hot spots," cor-

75

respond directly to significant points in acupuncture. I believe that people who have FM have a tremendous amount of internal energy (or *chi*) that tends to get stuck. Some *tai chi* teachers require extremely low stances that are not good for people in pain. One such pose, called the "holding posture," is good for the general student, but the holding posture is not good for people who have FM.

Try to find a teacher who has specific experience in teaching classes for people with special needs. I think that when people go to a *tai chi* instructor, they need to tell the teacher what their limitations are. Tell the teacher up front, "I have FM" or "I have CFS." Tell the teacher that you cannot or do not want to do the holding posture or other postures that bother you. You can gently step out of the posture or bring a little bit of movement into your body instead of holding a posture steadily, so you are not in a static position. There are many different types of teachers, so try to find a teacher who is interested in teaching *tai chi* as a way of health rather than as a workout.

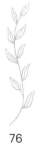

Chapter 6

Mental Health and Spirituality

I T'S IMPORTANT for us to remember that we must give as much attention to our mental and spiritual health as we give to our physical health. In this chapter, you will find numerous techniques that will help you deal with the mental-health and spiritual aspects of FM and CFS. It should not be considered a sign of weakness to seek mental health, psychological, or spiritual counseling during this time, especially if you have been newly diagnosed. In fact, therapy for these often-overlooked aspects of chronic illness is becoming more widely accepted.

Many physicians and psychiatrists believe there is not much of an organic basis for FM or CFS; instead, they believe that depression and anxiety may be at the root of these problems. They think that FM and CFS are simply somatic or physical manifestations of depression, rather than thinking of depression as a symptom of the syndromes. Patients often run up against this attitude, and they may come away from a visit with a practitioner feeling that the illness is all in their minds. But, in fact, quite a bit of information now suggests that FM and CFS have a more biological basis.

One of the reasons this myth exists is that one main treatment approach used in FM (at least in standard Western medicine) employs medicines that are also used as antidepressants. These medications help to normalize neurotransmitters in people with FM or CFS. Current theory holds that the medications work via this normalization, not necessarily because they affect depression in any particular way.

Regardless of the basis for FM and CFS, many of us are beginning to realize how profoundly our illnesses have affected our emotional and spiritual lives. Betty M., for example, says that having FM and CFS has radically changed her life. Before her diagnosis, she pretty much took her health for granted. After the diagnosis, she felt as though her body had betrayed her. She had a very difficult time dealing with this.

Betty had to quit her job before she even knew what was wrong with her. "I was in so much pain from my feet that I was becoming more and more exhausted. I began to have pain all over. Then I received the diagnosis of FM. I'd never even heard the word before. My podiatrist, of all people, guessed at a diagnosis and sent me to see a rheumatologist specializing in FM treatment. During the week between appointments, I was so scared, thinking that this FM thing was going to kill me! This is a good example of where I was mentally—depressed and scared beyond words." After years of talk therapy, Betty came to realize that she had to find a place inside herself to make peace with all the things that had happened in her life—including her chronic illness.

"Also, having to deal with the state Department of Social and Health Services [DSHS] for my meager monthly allowance, haggling with Social Security to get disability benefits, and struggling to get by financially had worn me down—mentally, physically, and spiritually. The anxiety of the unknown—whether I would continue to get welfare benefits, whether I would be able to get Social Security benefits, whether I would ever be able to work again, whether I would be sick for the rest of my life—was almost too much to bear emotionally. I became very depressed," Betty says. "Although I had suffered from depression my entire life, I was able to control it with medication and counseling. But this was a catastrophic feeling of loss and despair. I felt like I had no reason to get out of bed in the morning. My whole identity had been wrapped up in my job, and now my job was being a full-time patient."

Sometimes denial and self-blame can be issues, too, as David A. points out. "There's a lot of denial. 'Did I choose the wrong career? Is it something I did? Did I have the wrong attitude? Did I take care of myself? If I had, maybe I wouldn't have gotten this.' My FM came on so slowly over a period of years that as each new thing afflicted me, I'd go through anxiety all over again. First it was the hands, then migraines, then mental issues—lack of clarity, confusion, and short-term memory loss."

Ellen J., who has CFS and FM, says, "I have intermittent depression that comes from trying to cope with chronic illness. I know I'm really fatigued if I'm so tired that I can't even feel good about life. I looked in my journal from 1997, and I saw that I had only five days that year when I had no pain, and less than twenty days when my pain was even barely tolerable."

But like many people with chronic illness, Ellen has learned to rely on those around her. "Luckily, my support network is pretty good. I have a lot of good friends and family, although most of my family lives in other states, and most of my friends are people who are sick with various things, too. I moved to go to school, away from my old support network. And I haven't been well enough to be out where well people tend to be. I have health-care providers who assist me on a regular basis. I work on spirituality and academic interests, and I've made some Internet contacts."

Barbara M.'s FM and CFS cause her a good deal of mental anguish, too. "Some days I wonder how I can set a date for my wedding when I could wake up feeling just awful that day, and how I can get through the wedding. Days like that are really depressing, and when I have too many of them in a row, I get pretty down," she says. "I just can't pick a date a week from now, or even a few days from now, and say, 'I'm going to do this, this, and this,' because I might not be able to. One of the biggest changes being ill has made in my life is that I've spent my whole adult life *not* planning for the future.

"My main support network is my fiancé, but I try not to complain too much because I think it gets kind of boring," Barbara says. "I just set my own schedule, and even if I'd meant to go out into the world today, if I don't feel good when I wake up, I stay at home and try to get what I can done there."

People who have lost their health, their jobs, and, in some cases, their sanity find that relationships with friends, family members, and significant others become more important than ever. Friendship feeds the soul. Ironically, we sick people have the hardest time keeping friends just when we need them the most. When people become disabled, they simply don't have as much energy to spend on maintaining relationships. If a healthy friend isn't willing to give a little extra to make up the difference, that friendship isn't going to survive. Perhaps since they are not ill themselves, these people might not even recognize that a little effort goes a long way. Simple gestures—like offering to drive a person to the doctor, calling after a particularly difficult week, or offering to do a household chore—can make all the difference in the world. Long-term close friendships are like marriages: they should be for better or for worse. Unfortunately, we live in a disposable culture; oftentimes, the injured person gets "divorced."

Many people don't know how to relate to a sick person; they are uncomfortable and don't know how to be with a person who has changed so drastically. "My illness progressed over a period of several years," Mari says. "When I had to give up my job, I lost friends." She felt lonely because she wasn't working and her friends all had to work during the day. "I can understand it. I just wasn't as much fun as I used to be. Some people did pull away."

Andrea had similar experiences. "I felt like I had been abandoned," she says. "I always considered myself a good friend—if someone needed anything from me, buddy, I was there for them. I used to have dozens of friends, but at the very time in my life that I needed them most, they just weren't around."

Barbara M. says, "Basically, I don't tell anyone that I'm ill. Very few friends know. I've told people that I have headaches and stuff, but I don't go around saying, 'I have FM, I have CFS.' I just cope with it. If you were to ask my friends, they'd say I'm very hard-working, happy, and positive. Nobody sees me when I'm not feeling well, because I don't go out in the world."

Ellen J. says, "My siblings are supportive, but they just don't get what my illness is like on a day-to-day basis. And I guess they think I'm just sitting back and collecting disability rather than going to work. But most people who have known me over time saw me change and were really good friends; they have stuck with me and tried to help me cope with the changes that I've gone through."

Dealing with family problems can add to our stress. Sharon W. says, "If there's a lot going on in my life, and there always is, I can't just cut out the stress. My daughter's a drug addict, and she's gone. I'm raising my two grandsons, and their dad's a recovering addict. He is doing well and he means well, but he isn't mentally fully mature yet. And my mom is dying; she's got cancer. My grandson Nicholas has just hit the teen years, and the younger boy has attention-deficit disorder. My husband has a potentially deadly disease. So when they say, 'Try and stay away from stress,' that's a laugh."

Intimate relationships, too, can be difficult during chronic illness. For example, Andrew M., who has FM, says, "Right now, I'm not even dating. I haven't been seeking or been open to any kind of a relationship. Actually, if I met somebody and I thought there was a chance of a relationship, I'd probably turn and run the other way. I've been celibate for twelve years now. I would like a significant relationship with someone, but I look at myself as 'damaged goods.' I can't really take on a job or fulfill my half of the bargain, although now that I have disability income, I could probably support myself. My life is very limited. It's going to take a special kind of person to want to be in a relationship with a person who has these limitations."

Annie D., who developed FM after a car accident, points out that the physical pain of illness can be just the beginning of our troubles. "Hurting on a daily basis isn't bad enough; we get fired from our jobs, we are denied medications, and we are expected to just deal with it. Physicians tell you that you can no longer work. But if you don't work, how does the rent get paid? You struggle as long as you can to get by without any sort of income at all, no help at all. [If you're involved in litigation and consider a return to work], your attorney will tell you that it will be used as proof that you can work, that you aren't injured, that you've been lying all along.

"Before the accident, before FM, before doctors' visits and sixteen-pill-days, I always based my decisions on whether I would regret them later. As they say, you don't regret the things you did; you regret the things you didn't do. Now and forevermore, I will carry with me at least one regret: that I was traveling in the left-hand lane that fateful day. I will regret it for the rest of my pain-filled life."

Occasionally, even doctors can add to our troubles. Sharon W. says, "The first thing the doctor wants to do is drug you. But I just can't take drugs. People will try to tell you that if you just took a bunch of tranquilizers, you'd be all right. I'm finding that you've got to watch doctors. They get busy and can't keep up on their reading. The fact that you go to doctors for help and some of them don't even know what they're doing is the biggest joke of all to me. I do mostly natural remedies now. Especially since my hysterectomy, I can't even take a normal antibiotic without for sure getting a yeast infection."

Coping mechanisms vary among the people whom we interviewed for this book. FM patient Linda Martinson says that writing poetry has become her best coping strategy. She has published a collection, *Poetry of Pain* (see Bibliography). "In the beginning, support groups were very important to me. I could meet other people who had the same illness, who understood, and I would always leave a meeting energized," she says. "The focus was positive in those groups, not despondent. But then I found that writing helped fill a need in me that nothing else can.

"There's a poem in my book called 'The Yearning,' where I talk about how sad I am that I can't lay my head on my husband's chest anymore. I used to cuddle up there and go to sleep, but I can't because my neck hurts too much. It's just heartbreaking. When I read the poem at a conference, a woman came up to me with tears in her eyes and told me, 'My husband sleeps in another bedroom now. He is so afraid to disturb me. I want a copy to give to him because it breaks my heart that we don't sleep together.' Another woman said, 'I really miss the sexual relationship with my husband. My libido is really blah now.' It *is* something that we miss, because a loving sex life draws you closer together in your marriage or relationship. Marriages either break up when a spouse has a chronic illness, or the partners get closer."

Fifty-nine-year-old Sherry J., who is married with three children, says, "How does a person cope with FM? Ha! I am the leader of a FM support group, and that helps. I've learned to just say no. I have to limit my life. In other words, I live in a little box. That's the way I cope with FM. I have a network of friends. I have a great support group. Not that it's great because of me—it's great because there are some great people in it.

"Two years ago, I took care of my three grandchildren for eighteen months. There I was, at fifty-seven years old, raising three teenagers! How I ever did it, I don't know. But anyone who meets the children will tell you that they are fantastic."

Sharon W. says that in her search for an FM diagnosis, she went to an immunologist who told her, "This is all in your head; you need to see a psychiatrist." She says, "I found myself feeling like I was living in somebody else's skin, like I was going crazy because I was on straight Premarin [an estrogen replacement therapy] and had no testosterone in my body. I caught myself one evening with the knife pressed to my stomach, leaning against the sink. Something snapped, and I was past even caring if the boys found me or anything. I was a mess. I went to my general practitioner and told him how I felt. He gave me a shot of testosterone, and the difference was just amazing. I felt normal again.

"I pay much more attention to what my body is doing now, not only because of the FM, but because I had a hysterectomy and it threw me into instant menopause. Those symptoms have not gone away, and they're not likely to. You can get real sick of being sick, but you have to just do things anyway. Hurting or not, I'm going to do things anyway."

■ ■ ■

Having a chronic illness can make a person totally alter their belief systems, too. A religious person could start questioning why God has allowed them to suffer so. An atheist might start praying for relief. People who were once independent and strong-willed suddenly find themselves dependent and weak. People who always depended on others are suddenly forced to look inside themselves for the strength to go on. Sometimes, when everything else has been taken away, relationships are the only thing that can sustain a sick person.

Mari says that when she found her support group, she found herself surrounded by people who were going through the same thing themselves, who accepted her friendship "as is." Here were people, she says, who had the same condition that she did, and she felt so much comfort in knowing this. Eventually, she realized that everything that happens, happens for a reason. She tried to discover what lessons she was meant to learn from her illness. Mari says that she never had a "faith" or organized religion before February 1996, when she attended a women's purifying ritual for the New Year. That night, she says, she felt connected, a small part of the entire world. After that experience, she began attending regular rituals and cofounded a new women's group. She says it's filled a giant hole in her spirit that she didn't even know she had.

Her most spirit-altering experience came after she injured herself about six months ago. She was lying on the sofa in great pain and began saying a healing prayer. At that moment, she says, she experienced an amazing, healing love that she recognized as Jesus Christ. She felt a presence that held her and filled the room. "I knew then that no matter the name of the healer or the type of religion, no matter whether it's God or the Source that you believe in, suffering is, in my opinion, universal, and healing of the spirit is possible," she says. For the first time in her life, she truly understood the words "mind/body/spirit connection."

Emotional and spiritual healing can come gradually, too. Ellen J. says, "I've been living with FM for six years now. I'm no longer bedridden, although there are days that I do spend in bed. At this point, I am between forty or fifty percent of what I was before I became sick, which is better than ten percent (I still have trouble doing heavy cleaning, shopping, and cooking). I get together with friends, I go to a support group, I go to medical appointments. I play my piano and I hang out with my pet rabbit. I'm not suicidal or depressed anymore. Even if I don't get any better than I am now, I'm finally at a point where I understand my condition well enough and can ride out the bad times and live with it."

Sharon W. says that one of the biggest drawbacks of having FM or CFS is that you get so busy concentrating on how to handle life on a day-to-day basis that you can't concentrate on spiritual matters. "I've been too busy with other things that have been changing in my life to think about how being sick is changing [my spirituality]."

Sherry J., on the other hand, has found that her illness has given her a greater spiritual focus: "Being sick my whole life has meant that I never had time to think about God. I was always a Christian and lived a Christian life, or tried very hard to, but I didn't go to church. I couldn't have made it this far without God. I have no doubt that there's someone much more powerful than I am. I don't really pray, but I try to give as much as I can. That's my way, and it comes back in return. I now believe that God is inside us, and we each have our own ability to believe and be good and do good, or we can go the other way. Usually, if we go the other way, we pay for it. Whatever we give out, we get back. It's been proven to me over and over again in my life, with my grandchildren, my children, my illness, everything."

Illness can bring great transformations in our emotional and spiritual lives, some of them positive. For almost three years after the auto accident that caused her FM, Andrea allowed herself to wallow in self-pity and depression. She wandered around in a daze, wondering, "Why me?" She was angry and upset that something so catastrophic could happen to her. One day, she ran into an acquaintance at the grocery store. His hair was gone, and he had scars all over his head. He looked like he, too, had been chewed up in a car accident. She asked him what had happened. He replied, "Brain cancer." He had had a mas-

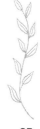

sive operation to remove malignant tumors from his brain. She expressed her sympathy and gave him a hug. As he turned to leave, he looked Andrea right in the eye and said, "Count your blessings."

Andrea says she did just that with every step she took on the way home that day. She gave thanks for her boyfriend, her girlfriends, the fact that she hadn't been paralyzed or horribly disfigured in the accident, the fact that she could still see and hear and smell and taste and experience this incredible universe. Since then, she's taken time out of every day to remember things to be thankful for. She is much more appreciative of a beautiful sunset, a barbecue, a cold beer, a silly program on television.

And the very accident that caused her so much pain and suffering also served as the catalyst for getting this book published. Andrea had been trying for years to get a novel of her own published; in fact, she had been working on the final chapters at the time of the accident. After she was hit, she completely stopped working on the novel. Slowly, she's come to accept what happened to her, and she's even perversely thankful that it happened—had it not, you might not be reading this now. And although she used to be bitter and resentful, Andrea now tries to use that energy toward more positive ways of living.

Ellen J.'s illness has helped put her more in tune with the universe. "I try to use my condition as a way to connect with the source, rather than feeling like I've been abandoned by something. And my spiritual practices have really changed. I found that I could no longer go to services, so that forced me to find other ways to be spiritual, including meditation, getting together with other women, and doing women's rituals. And also connecting with people on a nonsuperficial level, in contrast to how I think most people in our society deal with one another. I feel really blessed that I've had the opportunity to connect with people on a deeper level. I probably wouldn't have had this opportunity had I not become ill. I've had to examine who I am, whether my life is going in the direction it should go. Even though I would not have chosen to live my life in pain, I'm finally at peace with it."

Annie D. says she isn't at peace at all; she's downright angry. "I'd like a few answers from The Man and Woman Upstairs. How could my employer fire me when I could no longer work full-time? Aren't there laws against that kind of thing? No, because I had signed an 'at-will' agreement, which said I could be terminated for any reason at any time. Why was I allowed to suffer so much pain, and why did I have to wait so long to receive pain medication? Why was I prescribed nothing but anti-inflammatories that didn't help? Why did I have to beg my physician—five months after my accident—just to have an X-ray of my neck taken?

"Why did the woman who hit me just drive away, while I'm damaged goods for the rest of my life? Why do I have to wait years to find out whether I will be eligible for Social Security disability benefits? Why is my private disability insurance company allowed to drag out my claim year after year, in hopes that I will either give up or die? I worked to put myself through college, hustled to get myself better jobs, and set high career goals, so why am I now living in poverty?"

Andrew M. says, "Lately, I've been wondering more about the spiritual part of my life. I feel a need to have an active spiritual life. I feel a definite calling toward that. I think it would help me look at FM differently. One of the things that helped me most is the book *Full Catastrophe Living*, by Jon Kabat-Zinn [see Bibliography], because it talks about spiritual issues and how they relate to healing.

"I don't think I can give up hope that my FM will go into remission," Andrew says. "If I do that, I'll set myself up for having a problem with depression again. Some days, hope is all I have. To feel like there's no hope is the most disabling thing of all."

In addition to having hope, Andrea recommends that you get your very own theme song. Andrea's song is the Joe Cocker version of "You Can Leave Your Hat On," because she can jump and wiggle and sing at the top of her lungs. She puts her hat on, dances around, and doesn't worry about looking silly. This never fails to make her feel better. Some good theme songs are "Touch of Grey" by the Grateful Dead, Elton John's "I'm Still Standing," and the Eagles' "Already Gone." There's a beautiful song by George Harrison, "Heart and Soul." Of course, nothing beats Gloria Gaynor's disco hit "I Will Survive," or Queen's "We Are the Champions."

87

To help you get through your own times of despair and hopelessness, Andrea shares some other tips that help when she is down:

- Institute your very own "Diva Day." Go to a second-hand clothing store and buy yourself the ugliest, gaudiest, most polyester-filled gown (or suit) and tacky costume jewelry you can find. Complete the outfit with a rhinestone tiara and scepter (available at any costume supply company). On the days you're feeling especially bad, put on your diva drag. Swish around the house in fluffy mules, waving your scepter and practicing your queenly wave. Give yourself a name like Diva Foraday. (Andrea and a friend did this on days when they were really down, and it never failed to lift their spirits.)

- Laugh loud, laugh long, laugh often (see above). The French philosopher Voltaire once said that the art of medicine consists of "amusing the patient while nature cures the disease."

- Even if you're hurting so badly that you can't think straight, try to do one thing a day that makes you happy.

- Try to get some exercise, even if it's just a walk around the block or pulling a few weeds. Stretching and light yoga help ease aching muscles and can be done every day with little strain on the body.

- Listen to music you enjoy, or try new radio stations for a change.

- Visit your local library—it's crammed full of free books, videos, CDs, records, and information on community resources.

- Attend a book reading. Many of these are free or low cost.

- Splurge on bubble bath or bath salts (the ones that promote circulation and ease muscle tension) and enjoy a long, hot bath.

- If you can afford it, join a swim club. Water aerobics, swimming laps, hot tubs, and wet or dry saunas also help relax cramping muscles. There are community pools that are low cost or even free to use.

- Schedule an afternoon in bed now and then, just resting and watching videos.

- Eat a big scoop of ice cream occasionally, and don't sweat the fat grams.

- Grow a vegetable garden. Not only is this good exercise when done in small increments, but nothing is more life-affirming than producing and eating your own food.

- Find a charity and donate a few hours when you can. It will do more than benefit a worthy cause—it will give you the opportunity to focus on something other than your pain.

As Annie D. says, "I refuse to give up. Neither should anyone else. I won't roll over and suffer in silence. Most FM patients are women, and God knows women are experienced at suffering in silence. We've been socialized to believe that we have to work full-time, do all the grocery shopping, food preparation and clean-up, wash, dry, fold, and put away the laundry, and raise the children—all in the same day. Your first assignment as an FM or CFS patient is to give that up, sister, and give it up now. Also, if your doctor isn't taking your complaints seriously or won't prescribe pain medications, find another who will. Seek out treatment providers who specialize in treating FM and CFS. If you don't get relief from one kind of therapy, be willing to try another. If your friends don't make an effort to understand and sympathize with your situation, find others who will. Fight your HMO on every denial, especially when it refuses to cover expensive medications. Question authority. Read books. Join a support group. Your sanity depends on it.

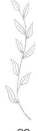

"Fight the 'poor-me' syndrome with all your might. It's easy to slip into that mind-set, and it *is* justified, since we feel so godawful bad most of the time. But it is ultimately a self-fulfilling prophecy—if you think you're pitiful, others will think you're pitiful, too. Whenever I'm feeling sorry for myself, invariably I come across someone who has it worse than I do. Once, I was at Kinko's, making copies of medical bills for yet another welfare application and feeling miserable. I looked up and saw a man who had obviously been burned in a horrible accident. He had thick scars and evidence of skin grafts and damage all over his body. One of his hands was completely burned off. My eyes teared up to think of the awful pain he must have endured. Yet there he was, carrying on his business like nothing was wrong.

"Examples like these never fail to inspire me to count a few blessings on the way home. Yes, I hurt, but I'm not paralyzed or terminally ill. Yes, there is no cure, but there are medications and therapies that make it more bearable. Yes, there are days when nothing seems to matter, but there are some good days, too. Yes, my situation is bad, but it could *always* be worse."

There are forces in the universe beyond our control—that's a lesson so hard for us puny humans to learn. For us, honoring our spirits means letting go of the need to control absolutely every aspect of our lives. This poses a special challenge for the stereotypical type-A FM personality, who's used to doing eighteen things at once. Every day, we may try to let go of the things that we know are totally beyond our control—yet there we are, expending precious energy trying to wrestle them into submission anyway. Having a chronic illness is a daily test of one's faith, and in this chapter, we'll show you some new ideas for passing that test.

Psychotherapy and Chronic Illness

Maureen Sweeny Romain

Maureen Sweeny Romain, M.A., CMHC, is a psychotherapist in private practice in Bellingham, Washington. Maureen specializes in counseling people with chronic illnesses and has recently added homeopathy to her treatments. She holds a master's degree in psychotherapy and spent nine years at the Fred Hutchinson Cancer Research Center in Seattle, working with patients who were receiving experimental treatments, and their families.

There are things you can do, psychologically, emotionally, and physically, to help your body heal. I work from the perspective that our bodies are really designed for health. Western medicine tends to focus solely on the disease, and in some aspects it does an absolutely wonderful job of curing disease. But it disregards the Eastern-medicine approach, which trusts the body's wisdom and ability to heal itself. In my practice, I try to find psychological, emotional, and spiritual places that support physical healing, particularly when I'm working with people who have FM and CFS or complications from cancer treatments.

There are different kinds of psychotherapy, and a person needs to search for a good relationship with a therapist rather than seeking out a particular type of therapy. If a therapist pays attention in that first session to how the person is responding, if a person has a sense of comfort or feels, "This is somebody I could develop a relationship with," that is more important than any particular technique that the therapist uses or any school of thought that the therapist follows. In fact, it's been found that regardless of a therapist's orientation, 70 percent of the people who go into therapy get better. So it's not like one therapy is better than others. (However, in some specific situations, such as phobias, there are particular therapies that are very helpful.)

Most therapists take some form of history from their clients to get a sense of where a client is coming from. Not just "I was born in a log cabin," but what their experiences in life have been, the significant experiences, good and bad, and the makeup of the client's family and support systems. It is important, too, to learn what the client expects to get out of the sessions. Sometimes, a client can't articulate that very well, but I think a therapist needs to ask this question: "How is it that you would like me to help you in this?" Therapy must be entered into as a collaborative effort between the client and the therapist.

I use a lot of different techniques. Particularly with people who have chronic illnesses, I look at what emotional and psychological baggage or unrealistic expectations they may be carrying. Now, just because you have some unresolved issue in your life doesn't necessarily mean that it causes your chronic illness or pain. But if your expectations are not being met, that can divert your body's energy, which is needed to help heal your problem. And so you're not using all that you can to help the healing process. It's helpful for people to work on this and let go, to surrender to whatever is happening in their life. That allows them to move on, to adjust the expectations that cause hurt and pain and sadness and dread, and to be able to focus on health.

One technique I use when working with clients on this issue is asking an individual to meditate on a particular word or phrase during the week between appointments. Examples are "humility," "surrender," or "let go of anger and want." They spend time thinking, being present with, and watching where this particular concept presents itself to them during the week. Often, the word or idea I suggest comes from what we talk about in session. Individuals are encouraged to do this with *mindfulness*, which is a Buddhist term implying great awareness. Some individuals have found this to be a powerful exercise.

Mindfulness just means having a level of awareness that allows you to use yourself as a source of information, helps you to make your way through this world. We're not often taught to operate in a mindful way, to look at our thoughts and feelings and what our bodies tell us about how we are doing.

This has led me to the belief that doing spiritual work can be an incredible healing force. I'm not talking, necessarily, about going to church, but rather about developing spiritual peace, about really connecting with a core part of ourselves that is about innate goodness and love. When we connect with that part of ourselves and live in that space (even momentarily), it puts our bodies back into balance. I believe this is challenging work, and we are increasingly seeing the importance of it.

Western medicine tends to look at only the physical aspects of the person and to address only physical symptoms. Yet it often misses emotional aspects, mind aspects, what people think, the beliefs that they hold, the perspectives or the frame of reference through which they view the world, and how these contribute to their well-being. In American society, too, we tend to go for the quick fix. If there's a pill for it, then I'll take it, and if one pill works, then golly, three pills might work better and quicker and faster. If you have a chronic illness, you are challenged to not necessarily go for the quick fix, but to work with your mind and thoughts and expectations. Also, you need to work on being grounded in your spiritual life. When you are working in all four of those areas, that's what healing is all about. A cure may or may not come, but emotional healing creates physical health.

Some people have hesitations about therapy. Part of the challenge is that we live in a society that puts a stigma on therapy and believes that you're somehow weak if you talk to a therapist. I've always believed that it makes less sense to *not* seek some consultation when you're struggling. If we break our ankle or have acute chest pains, it isn't considered a sign of weakness to go to the doctor, but when our psyches or our emotional selves are in pain, there's a social stigma on seeking help.

But we're increasingly seeing that paying attention to one's spiritual health is a very important component of healing. In the early days of cancer treatment, researchers found that women who went to support groups lived longer than women who didn't. The support groups may not necessarily have cured their disease, but these women lived longer and their quality of life was better than those who didn't attend. What they did was establish relationships with others, and that promoted the spiritual side of health.

■ A Patient's Story: Jill M.

Fifty-three-year-old Jill was living in Philadelphia, Pennsylvania, working for the Boeing Company when she was bitten by a tick and contracted Lyme disease. A small percentage of people infected with Lyme disease later develop FM, as Jill did. She and her husband (who works for Boeing, too) now live in Burien, Washington. She discusses how therapy helped her overcome the emotional difficulty that FM brought to her life.

At the time, I didn't even realize I'd been bitten by a tick. I was living with my second husband and my daughter, who was at the time going through a full-scale teenage rebellion. I was very ill one weekend, and I could barely crawl out of bed. But it went away, so I put it down to a forty-eight-hour bug. Six months later, I was getting more and more tired. My doctor ordered a "titer" test right away, and, sure enough, it came back positive for Lyme disease. That was the end of my life as I knew it.

I remember lying in bed watching a full two weeks of Wimbledon—all I could move was my head as the ball went over the net. I thought this thing would be over in a month or so and life would go on. I took massive antibiotics and coped with the resulting yeast infection, but there was little improvement. Of all the unlucky people who get Lyme disease—which in the mid-1990s was about 3,000 people in Pennsylvania and about three in Washington State—only 8 percent go on to develop FM, as I did.

I did not have to endure some of the horror stories I have heard from others as they made the rounds of disbelieving doctors. However, I did not have the faintest idea what my disease really meant. I was still fixated on Lyme disease. I thought life would go on normally, maybe a little slower, but essentially I would be the same person and would get better.

At that stage, denial was the order of the day. I went back to work, half-time for about three months and then full-time because I could not keep up with the workload on a part-time schedule. Then I crashed with a vengeance. I used up all my sick leave and went onto disability leave, which lasted six months at 80 percent pay. I finally made the decision to quit. They would have given me a pity job, since I had more than twenty years with the company and was the only female manager in the engineering department. But I don't take well to pity, and I couldn't stand the thought of dealing with people who had once known me as an effective, intelligent person.

I knew it was the right decision, because my stress levels decreased immediately and I was able to say goodbye to that part of my life. I don't think my husband had quite the same level of relief. He was hugely supportive and took care of me wonderfully, but I don't think either of us really understood that this was going to be a massive life change for both of us.

My major difficulties at this time were sleeping, widespread muscular pain, debilitating fatigue, and short-term memory loss. I took Flexeril for sleep, but I needed more and more of it, and I was doped up all day. I underwent psychological testing that confirmed my short-term memory loss and knocked about twelve points off my prior IQ level, which did not please me one bit. (How do they do that just by looking at inkblots?)

My doctor came up with a brand-new sleeping pill, Ambien, which worked like a dream and had no side effects on the following day. I felt as if I had gotten my brain back. I started warm-water-pool physical therapy classes, and they were wonderful. They got me back on my feet, and I started building up some muscle strength. I was feeling better.

So, here I was all day with nothing to do, an ideal situation in which to return to school. (Some of us never give up!) Not just any school, but Bryn Mawr, which had started a new program for us older types. I figured I could handle a couple of courses a semester and maybe even have some fun at the same time. Fun had been sadly lacking for quite a while.

My husband and I talked it over, and he promised to help with household stuff so that I could use all my available energy to study. The first semester was really hard, but it was fun. I met some neat people and managed to ace both my courses, Latin and English.

It all came apart in the second semester. My husband invented a helicopter for Boeing, but the company decided to build it in Seattle instead of Philadelphia. He basically disappeared, and so did all my support. He tried commuting, flying home every other weekend, but it just about killed him, and he slept all the time when he was at home anyway, so what was the point? I learned a lot about stress; I fell apart emotionally as well as physically. I tried to keep going at school, but I found myself having to relearn what I thought I had learned the day before. I dropped out. Another failure.

We decided to move to Seattle. This thoroughly shocked the children. I still hadn't figured out that I was sick, not just weak, but I knew instinctively to run away from stress, and I knew that I couldn't manage on my own. We moved into our new house in July 1994. The process of finding the house had taken three months. I developed a raging ear infection and finally found a local doctor to give me antibiotics. He told me to "get a life" when I kept bursting into tears.

Then I went to group therapy. There were six of us. We bared our souls, and I finally realized that my life had changed irrevocably. I had to learn to accept that change, and to recognize and accept myself as a changed person. I began to settle in and feel a bit better. I had a new doctor to give me medication and a counselor who taught me cognitive behavioral therapy and relaxation techniques. I learned to identify the things that caused me the greatest problems; unfortunately, one of them turned out to be people. They plain wear me out. I haven't been able to maintain any friendships with non-fibro people. It takes too much energy, and the return on the investment isn't worth the trouble.

About two years ago, I developed a severe rash on my hands, lost forty pounds, and lost muscle strength in my legs. I had dermatomyositis. It is a rare autoimmune disease; only one person in 300,000 has it. The cells in the muscles attack one another and gradually kill themselves off. Luckily, I had been diagnosed before any major damage had been done. (Incidentally, I had just applied for Social Security disability for my FM, and the diagnosis came through at the right time for a quick approval.)

Obviously, that was not a good year, and depression set in. The powers that be decided I should start drug therapy to counter the depression. Over the years, I had tried every depression drug on the market, as it is standard therapy for FM. I reacted badly to all of them. But new ones were available, so I tried one. I had a very bad central nervous system reaction. Instead of taking me off of it, my psychiatrist threw other drugs at me to tamp the reaction down until I finally said, "Enough."

By this time, my brain was a sponge and my heart did not want to live anymore. It was an astonishingly seductive experience: All I had to do was go to sleep, and there would be no more pain, no more fear, no more crushing fatigue, no more anxiety attacks. Just peace, beautiful peace. Even though I ultimately decided to choose life over death, I ended up spending four days in a psychiatric unit. What an experience. They sorted me out and sent me to a different psychiatrist who specializes in mixing drug cocktails for people like me.

While my life is not exactly a bowl of cherries, as my psychiatrist points out, I survived. With the dermatomyositis treatment regimen, which includes methotrexate and prednisone, my hands are considerably better. I am back in warm-water therapy and try to go twice a week; walking laps in a warm-water pool on a regular basis strengthens my leg muscles. I am still trying, but the setbacks come as regularly as the steps struggled forward. It is often difficult to maintain an upbeat frame of mind. But I try not to lapse into thinking that it's easier to do nothing.

I have found that my capacity for compassion has ballooned since I became ill. I can almost sense when others are in pain, mentally or otherwise, but I've had to learn that I do not have the capability to provide support. I need it too much myself, and I am too proud to ask for it. But I'm still on my path, and I haven't fallen off yet. Who knows what's around the corner? I accept that all these life events are straws upon a camel's back—each of us has a different camel; some are stronger, some weaker. My particular camel collided with a tick, and the tick won.

Spiritual Counseling and Chronic Illness

Cornelia Duryeé Moore

Cornelia is a thirty-nine-year-old actress who is studying to be an Episcopal priest. She works in the field of healing prayer and also has FM. She and her husband have two sons, and they live in Seattle, Washington. She believes that prayer can help heal those with chronic illness.

I have been a practicing Christian for twenty-five years. I became interested in healing prayer about fifteen years ago when I took a two-year course from a healing prayer counselor, Reverend Tilda Norberg. She teaches a course for ministers and others who work in counseling and want to learn how to pray for people in a healing way. She is a Methodist minister, one of the first female ministers ordained in this country. Her seminar sent me on a wonderful journey into healing.

Here's one example of how healing prayer has affected me and my family. I had been sick with FM, multiple chemical sensitivity, and endometriosis for some time. Before I got married, the doctors who had been taking care of my endometriosis said they did not think I would ever be able to conceive or carry a child. My friends and coworkers in healing prayer had an all-day prayer session for me—what they call "soaking prayer." Three women gathered around me as I lay just under the altar in the church. They prayed for me, they sang, they put their hands on my stomach for hours at a time. (They were praying for my fertility.) It was one of the most glorious times of prayer I have ever experienced. The women were so loving and so generous, and I felt that the Spirit of God was really there. My son was born two years after I was married. It was miraculous.

Soaking prayer can be one of two things. It can be a marathon session, like the one those women did for me. Or it can be praying day after day, week after week, just being in the presence of God and inviting God's will to come into your body. And miraculous things happen and the healing that takes place isn't always just physical. God's agenda may not be the same as ours. Healing can come in all sorts of forms. My agenda is not always dealt with in the way that I think but God's agenda always will be. God affects healing in our spirits and souls in addition to our physical bodies (or instead of, in some cases).

I recall many other examples of how healing prayer has been a blessing. Our family went through a terrible crisis two years ago. Within a two-week period, everything horrific that could happen did happen. I lost my seventh pregnancy, my husband was in a terrible accident, and we were fired from our jobs in the theater we had founded. The church gathered around us in a way that was holy, uplifting, and strengthening. We didn't have to cook for a month. They brought us food; they mowed our grass; they prayed with us and for us; they sent us notes every day to let us know they were thinking of us. It was the most beautiful outreach of the body of Christ that I have ever experienced, and it just blessed us down to our socks. In the midst of our terrible grief and pain, the church was like a dolphin swimming alongside another dolphin that is giving birth, helping to support it as the pain fades and a new life is born. It was a perfect example of how people in the church can be family to one another.

Currently there's a trend within the medical community to tend to patients' spiritual well-being as well as their physical needs. I know that nurses are learning all sorts of groundbreaking spiritual healing techniques, like laying on of hands, energy work, soaking prayer, all sorts of things. I've read that almost half of the nurses practicing today are doing this. That is just surprising and wonderful! Miracles of healing are happening every day.

My spiritual director gave me a prayer that has been very helpful as a centering prayer. Christians use centering prayer in the same way that Buddhists use mantras or other faiths use certain centering words or chants. It's an ancient prayer that has been used for almost two thousand years. You simply say "Lord Jesus Christ" as you breathe in, and "Have mercy on me" as you breathe out.

When I am in trouble, when I'm scared or upset, or have a nightmare, that prayer is the first thing that comes to my consciousness. It has become my default setting, if you will. It's very comforting to me, because I'm saying the name of the Lover of my soul over and over again. There's great power in saying His name, we Christians believe. It's very holy to me.

Some people just pray the word "Love" or "Peace." Anything that is holy to you or that pulls you into your experience of God can be used as a simple breathing prayer. It can be done daily in a ritualistic form. It can be done in traffic; it can be done in the bathroom; it can be done anywhere. It's lovely to have a subconscious prayer that happens almost without thought. Sometimes I burn a candle and use it as a centering device in my prayer. Some people hold a rock or something else from the earth. I think that women, especially, are very drawn to rituals and altars (which could be just pictures of loved ones). I always have an altar of central things in my room that focuses me. These things are icons of God to me. An icon, they say, is a window to heaven. Anything can be an icon for you and help you pray. It will change as you and your spiritual life change.

I believe that the Creator made us as a unity, as wholeness. The word "whole" comes from the same root as "holy," which also means "healthy," "hale," and "hearty." That is very significant to me. I think we are meant to have a sort of circle, a wholeness within ourselves, and that the spirit should not be ignored in any healing journey. Our spirits are very important parts of the package that makes us "us." If you ignore your spirit, it will send you dreams to tell you to be more sensitive. I believe one reason I am making such progress in my own healing is that my lovely Lord, my Holy Spirit, partner in my healing, will not let me ignore my spirit. I get these wonderful nudges that remind me to pray or to be mindful of God.

In their book *Stretch Out Your Hand: Exploring Healing Prayer* [see Bibliography], Tilda Norberg and Robert Webber define Christian healing as

> a process that involves the totality of our being—body, mind, emotion, spirit, and our social context. That directs us toward becoming the person God is calling us to be at every stage of our living and our dying. Whenever we are truly open to God, some kind of healing takes place, because God yearns to bring us to wholeness. Through prayer and the laying on of hands, through confession, anointing and the sacraments, and other means of grace, Jesus meets us in our brokenness and pain— and it is there that He loves, transforms, forgives, redeems, res-urrects, and heals us. Jesus does this in God's way, in God's time, and according to God's loving purpose for each person, because the Holy Spirit is continually at work in each of us, pushing us toward wholeness.

The process of healing is like removing sticks and leaves from a stream until the water runs clear. If we simply get out of the way of the Lord's work, we can trust that we will be led to the particular kind of wholeness God wills for us. Very often, the results of our healing are increased faith in God and a new empowerment to love and serve others. Frequently, we find that the very thing that caused our greatest brokenness becomes transformed into our own unique giftedness.

In this book, Tilda also reminds us what Christian healing is not:

> It is not magic. It is not manipulating God to do what we want. Rather, it is surrendering to God's healing work in us. Christian faith for healing is not a prediction of what God will do. It is simple trust that God loves us and is at work in us already. It is not proof that we are faithful or holy but, rather, a sign of God's love.

There's a great book on forgiveness as a pathway to healing that I highly recommend as part of a healing journey, *Forgive and Forget: Healing the Hurts We Don't Deserve*, by a minister named Lewis B. Smedes. A great book that teaches you how to pray is *Celebration of Discipline*, by Richard J. Foster. It's not just about prayer; it focuses on other pathways to healing as well. A book on mindful prayer and living in the moment is *Practicing His Presence*, by Brother Lawrence. It was written several hundred years ago, but it is still a classic on focusing your prayer. A good book on starting a healing prayer ministry in your church or place of worship is *Blessed to Be a Blessing*, by James K. Wagner. Lastly, I recommend *Food and Healing*, by Annemarie Colbin, and John Robbins and Jia Patton's *May All Be Fed: A Diet for a New World*, which helps you focus on spirituality, food, and healing.

To try healing prayer, you don't need to have a particular faith. You do have to believe in something bigger than yourself. Belief in a "loving higher power," or however God appears to you, is fine. As you pray, you can imagine that love is coming into you; you can imagine God's forgiveness or healing power washing over you.

And you do have to practice. It's like learning the piano—you have to do your five-finger exercises. You can't just suddenly play a sonata. It takes a while to develop openness to the spirit of God. People who are new to prayer sometimes find it helpful to focus on the word "God." You don't have to be very verbal about it; healing prayer is wonderful that way. I know one woman who had trouble with the idea of Jesus as a man, so she just imagined a large, beautiful dove bringing her the gifts of God. As you may know, the dove is a symbol of the Holy Spirit, so it worked really well for her. Imagery is very useful in healing prayer. Often, when I pray for a client, I see a little movie or a series of pictures about what is going on in that person. When I describe what I see to clients, they often are astounded because it seems like the Holy Spirit is talking to them.

You have to be humble, you have to be open, and you have to be receptive to whatever gift God sends to you. It's also important to have a sense of humor about it all. There's a beautiful passage in the Bible (Proverbs 17:22) that speaks to the need to keep a sense of humor through your hard times: "A merry heart doeth good like a medicine." Laughter can be blessedly healing, and keeping joy in our hearts is one of the keys to living a better life—for anyone, not just those with chronic illness. As author and theologian Madeleine L'Engle puts it: "Joy is the infallible sign of the presence of God."

If you are interested in finding a healing prayer group, just call a church in your area. Call some churches that sound good to you. Most Christian churches and some synagogues, too, have a prayer chain. It's a group of people who will put you in their daily prayers. I am an associate of a convent, the Community of the Holy Spirit in New York City. It is a great comfort to me to know that every day those women pray for me, and every day I pray for them. They are very holy women. Their job is prayer. That's what they do.

If you find a group who will pray for you, you don't necessarily have to "buy" their whole package or believe in their specific teaching. If you trust them enough to ask for their prayers, they will be honored to do it, because that is a call that all Christians share. That is true of other religions, too.

Come to God humbly and openly, and listen to the Holy Spirit instead of always giving God your list of desires. Listen to what God may have to say to you, present your request in a humble manner, and God will hear you. I don't think any prayer is ever wasted; every prayer is heard and answered. The answer may not be the answer that we would choose, but there is always an answer. There's always a change in ourselves and a blessing from God.

I think that healing prayer could be, for someone who is open to it, the single most important step toward recovery. I say that with knowledge of what I've seen happen in people's lives, and in my own life, when we're opened to the power of God. Exploring healing prayer could be a really great blessing to many people. It could bring a measure of wholeness that may be missing in your life.

A Patient's Story: Diane K.

Diane, forty-five, promotes and implements continuing education for acupuncturists. She is married and lives in Seattle, Washington. She has CFS and FM.

Having this illness has forced me to come to terms with what is important and what isn't. The mind/body connection is one of the things about CFS that's so important but so hard for people to come to terms with. I think we need to be more understanding about the connection, that one affects the other and that it's nothing to be ashamed of, it's not a bad thing. It's just the way it works. If you're having a lot of stress and if you have diabetes or CFS or whatever, it's going to get worse.

For some reason, we'll acknowledge that stress exacerbates asthma or something, but if we suggest that it exacerbates CFS, that's somehow shameful. I could see myself reacting that way; it made me afraid to ask questions of myself. It wasn't until I really saw what I was doing and shifted my perspective a little bit that I could ask those questions.

One thing that really turned me around was Dr. John Sarno's book

103

Healing Back Pain [see Bibliography]. I'd gone to see a friend of mine back East who had this incredible back problem. Just walking from the train to the parking lot, she had to stop and lie flat on her back on benches five or six times. That's how intense her back pain was. But she read this book, followed his advice, and instantly had no more back pain.

Dr. Sarno talks a lot about the mind/body connection. He goes into detail about the physiology perpetuating physical symptoms, as well as all of the beliefs that we adopt about our problems. After reading this, it seemed like I had focused on my physiology and my symptoms until I was just one big walking illness, and I was nothing but my CFS anymore. It was all I ever thought about; it was all I ever talked about. Every waking moment, I was assessing my symptoms and seeing what I had the energy to do. "If I stay up late, I'll feel horrible the next day. If I get up too *early*, I'll feel horrible the next day. Can't eat this or it'll give me this symptom. I'm allergic to that, so I can't have it. This drug gives me that problem." I had all of these beliefs about my illness that I had developed over a period of years. I had tons and tons of them—I could list them forever.

And so I decided to challenge a couple of my beliefs and see what happened. I stayed up late, and the next day I felt okay. I got up early a couple of times. When I realized that I *could* actually get up early, that led to going back to work. And I decided to take a nap in the middle of the day because I felt like it, not because I have CFS. I started challenging all these kinds of beliefs and found that I could do most of these things. That was a huge turning point for me, because I felt like I had some power. My life was back in my hands again.

And I decided, quite abruptly, to stop always thinking of myself in terms of my illness, to not immediately go to my illness as a reference point determining whether I could do anything. I decided to not blame everything on CFS when I couldn't find a word or misplaced something. I could say no to something because I plain old didn't feel like doing it, not because I had CFS.

That uncovered some kind of miracle in me: the beginning of getting well. And I consider myself well now and have been working for a couple of years. I feel strongly that the work I did—discovering joy and peace, engaging in quiet introspection, asking tough questions, not being afraid—was really the most important part of my recovery.

If I define myself as strong and powerful, even if I feel lousy at the moment, then I'm more powerful. That shift in perspective seemed to work miracles for me. I don't see myself as someone who's very sick anymore.

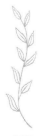

Chapter 7

Work and Vocational Therapy

THIS CHAPTER DISCUSSES the difficulties that sick people face when trying to find or keep a job. Issues such as workplace modification and vocational rehabilitation are explored in detail. For some people with FM or CFS, keeping a job is the one thing that helps them deal with their problem. Others are totally unable to function in a work situation. Helping both of these groups achieve their highest level of function with regard to work is one of the goals of this chapter. Before making any decisions about work, the reader is urged to make use of the many resources available (Web sites, libraries, bookstores, etc.) on the subject. In many states, local welfare offices have retraining programs for anyone who is reentering the work force.

After you've received a diagnosis of FM or CFS, making the decision to stay on the job or return to work is often an emotional one. Many of us go back to work not because we are well, but because we are bored or feel worthless when we do not work. Sitting at home by ourselves all day long, with no money coming in and unable to pay our bills, is no way to go through life. Sometimes we must choose another line of work that is very different from the one we were in before we got sick. With the loss of health comes the loss of financial security too.

Society defines people by their occupations. After you're introduced to a new person, the first question you're asked is, "What do you do for a living?" Answering this question honestly can be difficult, especially if you don't want people to know that you're not able to work or that you live on welfare. If you tell people that you don't work because you're sick, they may pity you or make a value judgment about your situation.

Ellen J., who has CFS and FM, says, "When I first became ill, I used to flinch when people asked me what I did for a living, because I was such a doer. I really defined myself by my job, by what board of directors I was on, what volunteer project I was working on. Over the last couple of years, I've really tried to change my focus from 'what I do' to 'who I am.' Who I am is okay, no matter what I do or don't do for work."

If you have made the decision to return to work, finding an employer willing to hire a chronically ill person is a long shot at best. Imagine that you are the owner of a small company. A prospective employee comes for an interview and tells you, "I have to have a special chair. I can only work twenty-two-and-a-half hours a week, and my computer has to have a special filter screen. I have to take a break every thirty minutes. I'm sick a lot, so I'll need to take lots of time off to go to the doctor. I can't tolerate any perfume or loud noises, and I get lots of migraine headaches. If I find that I can't do the work, I'll be applying for partial disability, so you'll have to fill out a lot of paperwork for me." Would you hire that person? Unlikely.

Many people interviewed for this book reported difficult adjustments after losing a job, reducing their work schedules, or having to leave school. Andrew M., for example, says, "I had been working as an electronics technician in the field for five years, covering five states.

Later I was in an office, helping other technicians who were on-site. [When I received my diagnosis,] I was angry, I was upset. I wanted to kill the messenger, not the message. To hear that I had something that there was no cure for and that they don't know a heck of a lot about didn't sit well with me.

"Shortly after I received the diagnosis, I lost my job. They said they were just letting a few people go—a reduction in the workforce. Actually, that's not what it was, but that's the reason my employers gave. They couldn't be honest and say they were letting me go because I had FM, because that would be something I could use against them legally."

Ellen J. says that before she became ill, she used to work sixty to eighty hours a week and went dancing two or three times a week. "I had a long-term relationship and did a lot of socializing. I enjoyed cooking and hosted a lot of dinner parties. I had what people describe as 'boundless energy.' I never had any trouble sleeping. After the chronic fatigue started in 1988, I could go for a while and then have to take four or five days to recover. It wasn't nearly as bad as when the FM kicked into high gear. I thought that I was just burned out on my job, so I decided to go to graduate school.

"I cut my workload down to forty hours a week and went to school at night to get my associate's degree in applied life sciences to prepare for medical school. I made the dean's list and did really well. I was also teaching classes and supervising doctoral students in clinical and community psychology. You could say I was pretty busy." After she began medical school, she found that "a full load in the summertime was eighteen hours, and during the regular school year it was thirty-two hours," she says. "I couldn't keep up. I had to leave that program."

Then, she says, "I was virtually bedridden for two or three years. I could get out of bed for very short periods of time to feed myself, heat up the heating pad, get a hot shower, and go to medical appointments. Other people had to help me with laundry and basic household chores. I couldn't drive that first year because my leg spasmed from sciatica and I couldn't hold the brake pedal reliably. I had to park it, literally."

Ann A., who once worked in accounting, tells us about her decision to leave her job: "I was having pain, but I was also experiencing one of the characteristic FM symptoms—'brain fog.' I had so much trouble doing the problem-solving things that you have to do with accounting. It scared the living daylights out of me because I was making significant mistakes with other people's money. I was dealing with megabucks in this job. I knew I needed to take some time off and recuperate.

"I thought I was only going to take three weeks off," Ann said, "but after a week and a half, I knew there was no way I was going back. I asked my replacement, 'Can you stay longer?' and he said yes. So I gave notice and quit, not knowing whether I was going to have any source of income. I had a private disability insurance policy that I thought would give me coverage, but I did not know for sure. I knew I couldn't continue working, because I was in horrendous pain."

Melinda N. experienced a similar crash-and-burn. She says, "I was a very busy woman. Dancer, author, seafood consultant, wife, mother. I was always an active person, taking on neighborhood causes, activities with my kids, activities at school. My husband is a commercial salmon fisherman, and I was in the fishermen's wives club auxiliary. I compiled a cookbook for that cause, and I lobbied as part of the West Coast Fishermen's Wives Coalition. Before my car accident, I did in-store cooking demonstrations as a seafood consultant. I was having a successful career as an author; I was on book promotional tours for months at a time. I was writing my second cookbook at the time of the accident. I wanted to continue my writing career, but it took me three years after the accident to write the third book in the series."

Now she worries that both of her two sons have lost their teenage years because she's had her hands full battling her FM. "My body was there, but the rest of me wasn't," she says.

Dennis H., an aerospace engineer with CFS, was at work when a supervisor committed suicide on the job. "That was a very stressful situation, and I had to take over some of his duties and deal with customer complaints. I believe that might have had something to do with my health deteriorating. I was seeing doctors and going to specialists, and I realized I wasn't going back to work any time soon.

"Quitting was a very difficult decision for me to make," Dennis says. "When you do something eight hours a day, five days a week, for as long as I did, you take a lot of pride in doing your job well. It feels like I stepped into an alternate universe. Being sick all the time requires a tremendous adjustment in your lifestyle. Dealing with it emotionally and psychologically is quite a challenge; in fact, it's almost a Catch-22 situation for me. I did a fairly good job of adjusting to what has happened, and I'm not letting myself fall into the depressive state that often happens after people lose their health and job and the activities they used to enjoy so much. I thought I stopped and smelled the flowers before I got sick, but I appreciate my health even more now."

Tom O. says that quitting isn't an option for him. "I've thought about it a lot, especially in the wintertime, when it's raining and snowing and I'm out there climbing poles. I'm thinking, 'I sure would like an office job.' But I've worked outside for so long, and I've been active for so long, I don't know if I could sit in an office eight hours a day, five days a week. I'm so close to retirement, a little less than eight years to go before I get a pension out of Ma Bell. After I get my retirement, I would like to continue with my photography, maybe get lucky and start selling pictures. If I won the lottery today, I'd be a volunteer for Children's Orthopedic Hospital. That's me, a future lottery winner."

Sharon W. says she doesn't have the luxury of not working, either, and cannot even consider working part-time. "When I turned forty (I'm fifty-three now), I realized that I couldn't get a new job as easily as I was able to before. I really had to work at it. I'm working in a deli now, which is a physically demanding job. There's a lot of heavy lifting, and you're on your feet all day. It means using your hands a lot, too. I've been here more than ten years. It's got good medical coverage, and because it's union, it's secure. And I have a good retirement plan, which is something I need, so I'm not likely to switch jobs anytime soon. I will stay with it until I can't physically manage it anymore; then I'll have to find a way out. I'm not trained for anything else."

Others have been able to create new opportunities for themselves. David A., who was working at Microsoft when he became sick, says that when he was diagnosed he didn't need to have a job right away, so he entered a graduate program and got an MBA. "The idea was to remove my dependency on my hands and create a new career for myself. I had a new focus; it wasn't like I was being forced out of my job and had nothing to do and no plan. At school, though, I had to constantly worry about where was I going to be, whether I could microwave my lunch or if I'd have to eat it cold. (I have to cook a lot of my own food.) I also have to choose activities on the basis of how quickly they will tire me out.

"But I completed the two-year program. Now I'm facing the reality of my new career and struggling with defining what I am going to do and how it's going to work. My wife is supporting both of us right now, and that's a lot of pressure on her because she feels like she can't quit, and we need the insurance for my health care. I have been fortunate in that I've had continuous health insurance and had a lot of money saved up before I became unable to work. I worry about whether I'll ever have an income that will support both of us and what my capabilities will be.

"I want to maintain a full professional career, to do great things in the environmental field. But right now, my professional ambitions are a lot smaller. They're more about getting a part-time job that pays reasonably well, being able to raise a family and maintain a household. My ambitions and my view of my potential in life are currently a lot smaller than they used to be. I hope this changes, but right now I'm trying to set realistic goals for myself and achieve those, rather than reeling in the big dreams."

Many people said that their relationships with coworkers were a deeply satisfying aspect of work—coworkers are like a family away from home. Losing this social support can be as devastating as losing a job. Before Erin P. was diagnosed, she had a great job at a software company. "I was meeting all kinds of people and being more social than I had been in a long time: exercising, hiking, you name it," she says. "I had all this energy and enthusiasm. Being diagnosed was sort of like getting struck with a bullet. I didn't understand what was going on. I had to quit my great job after about four years. I just couldn't do it

111

anymore. The longer I stayed there, the more I was draining myself."

Betty M. says, "The worst part about quitting my job was trying to explain to my family what was happening to me after I lost my livelihood, my freedom, my spontaneity, and the friendship of my coworkers. I couldn't adequately explain that it felt like my feet—my entire body, really—were on fire with a pain that I could neither explain nor escape." It seemed surreal to her to say that she had to quit her job because her feet hurt: "How insignificant it sounded."

For the person who is currently working, the need for workplace modification is a very real concern. You must be able to trust that your employer will be flexible enough to help you keep your job. A large corporation is a good option for people who are considering returning to work after illness, since they generally have policies in place that address people with special workplace-modification needs. These modifications could include an ergonomically designed workstation, job-sharing (in which two people work part-time in one full-time position), and avoiding prolonged standing or sitting. And it's important to avoid work situations that might further harm your health. Ann A. says, "Before I did accounting work, I used to work as an industrial hygienist, which is in the occupational safety and health field. We would assess workers' exposures to hazardous chemicals, and I was exposed to a lot of nasty stuff, too. They were short-term exposures, but I was repeatedly exposed just the same."

People can also negotiate for additional sick leave or vacation time that can be used to cover periods of illness or flare-up. Thanks to President Clinton's Family Leave Act, people can now take up to three months off work (without pay) to recuperate from an illness or care for a sick family member, without fear of losing their jobs.

Modified work schedules are possible for many people with FM and CFS. Diane K., for example, who has CFS and FM, says, "I've been working for a couple of years. I work four days a week. A couple of times I tried a five-day workweek, but I started getting symptoms and had to cut back again. Five days a week just doesn't work for me. Now my relapses have become farther apart, briefer, and less severe with fewer symptoms." Other people have not found much workplace flexibility. Sharon W., for example, says, "Because you look normal outwardly, people don't think you're sick. So if you have trouble doing something, you get comments about it. I finally took some information about FM to my bosses, but I still don't think they have any grasp of it."

People who feel that they are completely unable to function in a work setting may apply for Social Security disability benefits. Because of the different levels of disability among claimants, Social Security often has a hard time believing that people with FM or CFS are totally disabled and unable to work. Annie D. says that when she applied for benefits, she was denied twice. Even though Annie has a college education and enjoyed significant success in her career before she became ill—and despite the fact that all of her treatment providers had said she must avoid prolonged sitting and standing—the administrative law judge still ruled against her. In his decision, he wrote that Annie had an "unrealistically high expectation of herself" and could work as a convenience-store clerk, video security alarm monitor, or telephone solicitor. Annie said that she was insulted by the judge's remarks, and she felt worse after reading the decision than she did when she was fired from her job.

Many people also told us about lengthy struggles to procure disability and insurance benefits. Ellen J. says, "I've been wiped out financially. I live in subsidized housing for disabled people. I was very fortunate to get in. Because I used to be a social worker, it took me a while to get to the point where I could admit that I needed to be there. I applied for Social Security disability about a year into my illness, because it became clear that it wasn't going away, and I needed a long-term solution to deal with not having any money.

"It took four years from the time I got sick until the time I actually received benefits, three years into the application process. I had to get an attorney. I got my first check on my thirty-fifth birthday, which is also the same week I was supposed to have graduated from medical school. I'm also on Medicare and Medicaid. Medicaid is for people who are 'medically indigent,' which means my income isn't high enough to pay for all my medical costs. Because my medical costs are so high, my rent is also much lower. Each year, I fill out forms showing my medical costs—they take up about 80 percent of my income."

Some people have had an easier time getting benefits. Dennis H., for example, says, "I had a long-term disability policy through work. They sent out an insurance adjuster who talked to me about my health problems, my abilities and inabilities. I filled out a bunch of forms; they sent me to the company's doctor. I was approved for long-term disability coverage." And some aren't currently interested in disability benefits. David A. says, "I recently looked into disability insurance. There's not really a lot of helpful information out there, like a 'how-to-get-disability guide.' It feels like a declaration of the fact that I will never be a functioning member of society. I'm just not willing to take that step, so disability right now doesn't seem like an option."

People who say that you should just "get to work" do not realize that being ill is in itself a full-time job. Our days are spent managing our symptoms, making doctors' appointments, arranging for and picking up prescriptions, and going to acupuncture sessions. Sometimes, dealing with an HMO to get these things covered is harder than the jobs we did before we became ill. The current employment climate, with its downsizing, decreased job security, and employers who expect more work for less pay, makes it even more difficult for many chronically ill people to stay on the job or return to work.

When you're deciding whether to stay on the job or return to work, you must look for something that you really enjoy doing. Otherwise, work becomes too much work. Putting out lots of energy for a job you don't love is too draining. It's better to not work at all than to waste your energy in a no-win situation. Rebecca H., who has FM, offers an example. She worked at a hospital for six years before a bad shoulder forced her to quit. "Those twelve-hour shifts were so hard on my body," Rebecca says. "Waiting for the bus, I would want to sit down, but I knew I wouldn't be able to get back up again. I'm still a respiratory therapist, but during my bout with my shoulder, I was out of work for eighteen months. When I went back, I could only work eighteen hours a week, doing respiratory rehabilitation at a skilled nursing facility. In hospital work, you have a heavier caseload. In rehabilitation therapy, you only have two or three residents on your caseload. So you can sit and talk with them and do their treatment. You don't have to push ventilators or anything. That is much easier on my body."

Only you can judge your energy level and your real reasons for wanting to work. But if all you are able to do is go to work, come home, and crawl into bed and dread the next day, you have not made the right choice of employment. Jeopardizing your health for minimum wage doesn't help anyone, and it can actually make your situation worse. Finding a balance between working and healing requires a lot of soul-searching and effort. The rewards, however, can be worth the added stress work can bring.

Vocational Rehabilitation

Don Uslan

Don Uslan, M.A., MBA, is a psychotherapist, a rehabilitation counselor, and the owner of Northwest Counseling Associates, a private practice specializing in treating patients with chronic medical conditions and occupational problems. Mr. Uslan also cofounded the Center for Comprehensive Care, which provides rehabilitation services based on the philosophy that coordinated care will produce the best patient outcome.

Vocational rehabilitation is a term that's not well understood by the general population. Quite simply, a vocational rehabilitation plan helps support chronically ill people in maximizing their work potential. The treatment plan depends upon many variables: namely, the condition that a patient has, how they manage their life requirements while fulfilling their work requirements, and what changes can be made to make work fit into their whole treatment picture. Vocational rehabilitation also includes working with clients and their attorneys to allow the patient to work part-time, take time off work, go back to work, or change their work entirely if necessary.

115

A rehabilitation counselor may also work directly with employers, insurers, or other physicians by assisting them and providing information on other possible care interventions. The counselor may also make recommendations on legal issues such as disability benefits or reasonable modifications to a job or workstation. Vocational rehabilitation involves implementing plans that keep work part of the picture, and make receiving disability benefits a temporary part of the treatment plan as opposed to a long-term goal.

Should a person diagnosed with FM or CFS continue to work? Part of the answer depends upon what point of the treatment process you are talking about. Early on, people don't yet know what is happening to them. A year down the road, they may have a better sense of what's happening, and they are over the initial shock of being diagnosed with a chronic illness. Three or four years later, when they've had good treatment and are more experienced in managing their illness, work may be more appropriate.

Most people with FM or CFS require time off work to get themselves together, to focus, rest, and recuperate. Then they may go back to work. Speaking anecdotally, my impression is that only about 20 percent of the people diagnosed with FM can really stay on the job full-time. Even if circumstances are ideal, most people have a hard time functioning as employees in the current work environment. Usually, modifications are necessary. Some people are able to work out of their homes, which allows a lot more flexibility. Most others, though, have employers who are cooperative and can work with them.

It is hard for a person with FM or CFS to work a professional forty-hour workweek. Except for a very few situations, however, permanent disability is something I do not support. It does happen, usually when a good employer cannot be found or the patient has other responsibilities, such as young children. But work is good. Work is possible. And with proper employment strategies, in conjunction with good providers and treatment plans, people can expect to eventually return to a reduced work schedule. However, for a return to work to be successful, it requires soul-searching, adjustment, and coping with a major lifestyle alteration.

In 1989, I developed the treatment model now known as the Proactive Living Program. This sixteen-week group-model program is designed to integrate a variety of effective treatment approaches to save costs, allow greater communication among providers, and assist patients in gaining mastery over their medical conditions. The program provides adjustment counseling, including developing self-management strategies and skills for coping with lifestyle changes, support systems, goals, and relationships. The program also provides acupuncture, active-movement therapy, relaxation techniques, physical reactivation, and rehabilitation education (including occupational alternatives, disability issues, recovery planning, access to community resources, health education, nutrition, pain management, optimal sleep strategies, stress reduction, and pacing techniques). The program staff includes a nurse health educator, an acupuncturist, physical therapists, a medical psychotherapist and social worker, massage therapists, and medical specialty consultants.

A typical patient with FM who has gone through the program is Gwen [a fictitious name], a thirty-eight-year-old woman who was a claims examiner for a major insurance company. Gwen, who is married and the mother of two, had been recently promoted, but her growing fatigue, difficulty in concentrating, forgetfulness, and pain were adversely impacting her performance on the job. She struggled with FM for more than five years. During that time, she had nine physicians assessing her for a variety of medical ailments (including psychological conditions). Doctors thought Gwen exhibited symptoms of multiple sclerosis, cancer, tumors, and other illnesses. She spent thousands of dollars on a wide variety of prescribed medications and alternative herb therapies. At one point, one doctor suggested that she had FM but told her there was nothing to be done about it.

Finally, Gwen saw a good rheumatologist who referred her to the Proactive Living Program. Gwen met other people with similar conditions and began to realize she was not alone. While she learned about the history of her condition and what to expect from the future, she also began to experience some relief from acupuncture, careful stretching regimens, and specialized exercises. She learned how to monitor

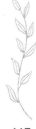

117

her symptoms and keep a diary. She learned techniques to help her sleep better, and gave her physician feedback about the effects of various medications. She developed skills in dealing with other people and their reactions to her. She learned the limits of her strength and energy, and how to pace her exertions.

Gwen informed her employer about her condition and gradually modified her work to two and a half days per week while supplementing her income with disability benefits. She decided to enter into psychotherapy to deal with some long-standing issues that caused her internal stress and anxiety. Stress-management techniques helped her to have periods of profound calm and served to generally "turn down the internal thermostat." Gwen learned how to cope with the flares and cycles of her condition. She formed close relationships with other group members and learned to rely more upon them and less upon health professionals.

A meeting with the program leaders and the group members helped Gwen's family members learn how they could help their loved one improve. Gwen began to feel increased self-confidence as she gradually gained some control over many of her symptoms. For the first time, she felt optimistic about the future. During the two or three years after she left the program, Gwen continued in a follow-up group and made gradual gains (with occasional setbacks), and she is now successfully working four days per week at her job. Her pain has decreased, her sleep is better, her concentration has improved, and she has gradually recovered energy.

Managing a chronic illness requires a strong support system. If everything is orchestrated correctly, I believe that patients can return to work (unless some other medical, physical, or psychological issues are going on). Many people who have been diagnosed with a chronic illness are in deep despair because they feel like they've lost everything. Our message is that it doesn't have to be that way.

Chapter 8

Natural Healing and Nutrition

T HIS CHAPTER ILLUSTRATES the principles of natural healing and introduces you to ways you can use them to fight FM and CFS. "Natural healing" refers to any regimen that reinforces the body's healing ability without relying on pharmaceutical drugs or surgery. Natural healing focuses on diet, herbal supplements, and vitamins as ways of helping the body return to its natural state of health. Diet can help purify the body and provide better nutritional support. Herbal supplements can bring about increased body function, while vitamin therapy can help replace lost nutrients. The combination of these three approaches will bring about the best possible outcome for the patient.

It is vitally important that people with FM and CFS maintain a good diet. Noted author Dr. Devin Starlanyl, along with the people we interviewed for this chapter, explains that our bodies are not as efficient at eliminating toxins as a healthy person's body, and so it is more crucial that we try to regulate the substances we put into our bodies. But this poses a special problem for us: we are so exhausted all the time that we do not feel like chopping vegetables, weighing portions, steaming rice, etc. (Andrea hopes she's not the only one who ever ate ravioli straight from the can!)

Lacking the energy needed for proper food preparation is something we fight on a daily basis. But since food supplies the body with energy, we're shooting ourselves in the foot by not meeting our special nutritional needs. Also, the typical American diet is by no means a healthy one. According to nutritionist Joleen Kelleher, digesting the normal American diet requires about 60 percent of the body's internal energy. "If you're only operating at 50 percent of your normal energy today," Joleen says, "and you have a normal American meal (which tends to be overcooked and overprocessed and contains a lot of sugar and red meat), it's going to take all of your energy just to digest your food."

But changing dietary habits requires a real commitment to feeling better. Humans are creatures of habit. If you grew up eating chicken-fried steak every Sunday, it's extremely difficult to give it up—even as it's coming back up. We eat when we're not hungry just to have something to do, or we don't eat at all because we're so tired. Food is a social activity throughout the world; we equate good times with good dinners, a good steak, or a good bowl of ice cream. We are prone to overeat or eat "no-no" foods in social situations. We know they're bad for us, yet at times we feel powerless to stop ourselves from having a serving (or two or three).

If there's any word in the English language (besides "exercise") more dreaded than D-I-E-T, Andrea doesn't know it. The avowed chocoholic in her just cringes when she hears that word, because it reminds her of when her parents forced her to go on diet after diet, beginning in the fourth grade. Andrea says she would watch her friends and family members enjoy her grandmother's homemade ice cream while she ate cottage cheese and hard-boiled eggs. She suffered through years of bulimic and anorexic behaviors before she was finally able to come to terms with her body weight, and she now realizes that since she's ill it's more important than ever to maintain a healthy diet.

Another dietary problem faced by people with FM and CFS is "stress eating." You know the feeling: your doctor's appointment was canceled even though no one bothered to call and tell you; the freeway was backed up as badly as your intestines; the dry cleaner ruined another pair of pants. The first thing you see when you walk in the door after this incredibly stressful day is the chocolate cake that then becomes dinner. Stress eating compounds our digestive problems in two ways: one, we've crammed our faces with junk; two, we haven't eaten anything nutritious.

So what exactly should a person with FM or CFS eat? Lots of fresh fruits and vegetables, along with fish or chicken (or a vegetarian protein alternative like tofu or beans and rice). Grains can be incorporated in moderation if you're not sensitive or allergic to them; however, carbohydrates should be limited in general. Processed foods should be eliminated as much as possible. Any kind of artificial chemicals or preservatives should be avoided. Red meat should be eaten in moderation, as should spicy foods. Some people have trouble eating a combination of foods in one meal; others have difficulty eating in a restaurant. Eating after 8 P.M. is discouraged. Excessive sugar and fat isn't good in anyone's diet, and this is especially true for people with FM and CFS.

Mari says, "I know I feel better when I eat healthy food on a regular basis. I try to eat a salad a day. I try not to eat much red meat. I'm trying to eat more fruit as well. But I'd be lying if I didn't admit that doughnuts and Pepsi are what I live for."

Jody E., a twenty-one-year-old student, eventually came to the realization that her diet needed to change when she started regurgitating her food due to excessive stress. "When it came to the point where I was immediately regurgitating everything I swallowed," she says, "I knew I had to make a change. I ate nothing but rice, Bartlett pears, and repulsive herbal tea for two weeks." Despite its restrictive nature, this elimination diet really helped her stomach problems. Ellen J. says that she takes a metabolic detoxification and stabilization nutritional product known as UltraClear Sustain, which uses white rice powder as its protein source [see Resources]. She's been on the program for

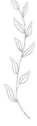

three years and has received a lot of benefit from it.

Erin P. signed up for a natural healing seminar at the Optimum Health Institute in San Diego, California [see Resources]. After three weeks on the nutrition-focused program, she felt remarkably better and her stomach problems were gone. She ate an all-raw-foods vegan diet, endured colon cleanses, and drank a lot of wheat-grass juice, but for her it was worth it. She now has her health back.

Irritable bowel syndrome and its nasty next-door neighbor, "leaky gut," along with nausea, constipation, and acid reflux, are many times part of the FM and CFS lifestyle. Rebecca H. has, among other things, irritable bowel syndrome. "My doctor told me I needed to eat 'closer to the earth,'" she says. "I went on a macrobiotic colon cleanse, and it helped tremendously. A simple colon cleanse is very easy to do. You cut out protein for about seven to ten days—all forms of protein, beans and everything. You give your intestines a rest by eating a lot of fresh vegetables and things like daikon radish, miso, and seaweed. They restore the normal flora in the intestines and actually heal them. So now I do a colon cleanse every year."

Becky R. has digestive problems, too. "It hasn't been labeled irritable bowel syndrome," she says, "but I'm working with a naturopath to identify some food allergies that affect my digestive system and cause me to not properly absorb what I'm eating. He says that if my digestive system is irritated and I don't absorb food, I could eat and eat and eat and not get any nutritional value or energy out of my food. That makes sense to me. So he's taking me off dairy, and we're going to try to eliminate wheat."

Andrew M., too, has had to radically alter his diet. "Dr. Devin Starlanyl's *Fibromyalgia and Chronic Myofascial Pain Syndrome: A Survival Manual* [see Bibliography] says that what seems to work best for people with FM is a diet that is made up of four parts carbohydrates, three parts oil, and three parts protein. I wasn't getting enough protein, so in the morning I have cereal and raisins, and I put powdered whey protein in the milk that I have with my cereal. That makes my breakfast feel like it lasts longer; I don't get as hungry as soon as I did before. I usually have only two meals a day and then I kind of snack.

I try to eat my big meals early in the day and my smaller meals or snacks late in the day. I need fruit, so I have that along with cottage cheese for a snack, or I make some rice and a bit of meat. I don't eat as many greens and vegetables as I'm supposed to, but I'm working on it."

Hilary S. says she is allergic to a lot of different foods and tries to stay away from them. "Sometimes I can't, though. I am especially allergic to wheat and dairy. Being more aware of what I am allergic to definitely helps me in terms of energy. But I do cheat. Sometimes I just *have* to have a bagel with cream cheese. I try not to overload."

Corrie M. has candida in addition to FM and CFS. Many of the symptoms of FM and CFS—joint and muscle pain, brain fog, memory loss, fatigue, endocrine troubles and sensitivities to mold, dust, and odors—can be mistaken for the symptoms of candida, which is an excessive growth of yeast in the body. People who are having FM or CFS symptoms are urged to be tested for candida, as their symptoms are remarkably similar. If candida is a problem for you, Corrie has this advice to offer: "The most important tool for managing my candida has been my diet. When I abstain from 'bad' fats and most animal protein and eat only 'good' oils and unrefined complex carbohydrates, I feel almost human." Corrie says she supplements her diet with *acidophilus* and *bifidus* [live cultures of beneficial bacteria found in yogurt and in the human intestinal tract] and stays away from known food and environmental allergens. "By rotating my food, supplementing with vitamins, and eating organically and lower on the food chain, I have actually recovered a small portion of my prediagnosis life," she says.

Naturopathy, in addition to nutrition, has helped many people whom we interviewed for this book. Sharon W. goes to a naturopath for hormonal balancing and takes numerous vitamins to help with her illness. "I've had a hysterectomy, so there are fewer natural hormones in my body," she says. "The FM got considerably worse after the hysterectomy. I went through a series of treatments, trying to get my hormones balanced; pills didn't work, so the doctor tried weekly hormone shots. When I reached a certain hormonal level, my FM pain stopped. The minute that level dropped, the pain increased again. It was a rollercoaster of

shots and pain, shots and pain. The problem with replacement therapy is that you can never duplicate the body's natural supply and demand. The hormones I'm taking have never stopped my hot flashes."

Sharon also suffers from arthritis. "I visit my naturopath on a weekly basis for physical therapy, and he uses heat and electrical stimulation," she says. "He has given me the most help. I asked him, 'What causes these arthritis attacks?' He told me that I retain fluid in my joints, and that barometric changes cause pressure and pain. He gave me a water pill that helped. I take three glucosamine tablets a day, 500 milligrams, which seems to alleviate symptoms, so that I'm at least mobile. Glucosamine replaces some of the materials your body normally makes that decrease after a certain age. If you quit taking it for about a month, you start feeling the pain again. I'm taking chondroitin and ginkgo biloba, too.

"I take one multivitamin and calcium daily. I take potassium gluconate, extra magnesium, and vitamin B-6 twice a day and 1000 milligrams of vitamin C three times a day. I take vitamin E twice a day, but not at night, because it can really disrupt my sleep. I use a selenium tablet at night, plus hormones and Estratest, along with a pseudo-progesterone cream made of wild yam. I'm really trying to cut back on the Estratest. I'm using the ginseng granules, and they give me a boost. There's a vitamin B-12 that you can put under your tongue, and it goes into your system faster than when you swallow it. That gives me a boost when I start feeling tired and droopy.

"All of this stuff is really expensive, and health insurance does not cover it. I spend more than a hundred dollars a month just on massage and the naturopath alone."

Over the years, the authors of this book have gone through a sort of trial-and-error process to help us identify problem foods. We've had to eliminate foods we can no longer tolerate, including the following:

■ tomatoes, white potatoes, eggplant, and peppers. (These can increase pain and may inhibit normal collagen repair in the joints or promote inflammatory degeneration of the joints.)

- peanuts and peanut butter (which can contribute to acid reflux)

- pizza (which can create intense heartburn and acid indigestion)

- dairy products (because of artificial hormones and pesticides)

- fried foods (for obvious reasons)

- spicy foods (which can inflame an already unhappy stomach lining)

And we've added these foods to help aid in digestion and for nutritional support:

- prunes and flaxseed oil (to help combat constipation)

- high-fiber cereal (ditto)

- coffee and a big bowl of oatmeal for breakfast (ditto)

- organic fruits and vegetables

This chapter provides many different ideas to help focus your attention on the importance of a proper diet. Radically altering lifelong eating habits takes a real desire to feel better. Every day, we should rededicate ourselves to the goal of better living through better nutrition. Pass the organic Cheez-Wiz, please!

Eating for Optimum Health

Joleen Kelleher

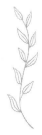

Joleen Kelleher, R.N., is director of the Light Institute for Health in Olga, Washington. This nonprofit organization teaches people how to make sustainable changes in habits that affect health. The institute focuses on changing habits of the mind, emotions, and physical body that prevent people from living life in harmony.

Nutrition is of utmost importance for anyone dealing with a chronic illness. Many care providers believe that nourishment of the physical self is as important as nourishment of the mental and spiritual body. When you see physical food as coming from nature, as alive and here to help produce harmony and the necessary nutrients for your body, your food becomes a reflection of how you nourish yourself spiritually. Our society does not reflect this. It has helped us move away from balance through advertising and fast-food restaurants. This has created a false belief that food is something other than nourishment, that we should eat it only as a social activity or because it tastes good.

Take the problem of lactose intolerance, for example. If you look at advertising, you see that you can buy a pill to take away your stomachache so that you can continue eating a particular dairy food. Many people are lactose intolerant, yet they take pills to mask the body's discomfort at having to process dairy foods. This illustrates how unconscious we are about the powerful nature of food. When we experience symptoms like feeling miserably overstuffed after a meal, that is the body telling us it is out of balance. It is not a meal the body can easily assimilate.

Awareness is critically important: awareness of the food we're taking in, of how that food is digested by the body, and of how the body feels after eating a particular food. Our bodies use food in two ways: for fuel and energy, and as the raw material the body uses to repair itself. When someone has a condition like CFS or FM, it is an indication that the body is very low on energy (on an internal "life force" level). I find that most people don't even have enough energy to digest their food.

One way that people with a chronic illness can heal is by increasing their internal energy. A bad diet will not help repair and heal the body. And the energy used for digesting that unhelpful diet is taken away from the energy the body needs for healing. One of the goals, then, is to prevent the energy the body needs for healing from being used up in digestion. We recommend two things to help fix this problem. One is fasting. Fasting frees up energy in your body so that it can help detoxify your system. That's one of the reasons why, at the end of a fast, people feel "lighter." They're actually feeling more energy, because energy has been freed and the body has been detoxified. The other solution is to simplify your diet, so that you're eating closer to nature and eating less processed food.

Fasting is an important aspect of healing from chronic illnesses. Lots of people are afraid of fasting because they think it is a kind of deprivation process, but it isn't. Rather, it is a way of resting the body while healing goes on. However, many people who fast inappropriately immediately go back to the way they ate before, at a time when the body is very vulnerable and hungry for new nutrition. If dirty feet walk across a clean carpet, it is more visible than when dirty feet walk across a dirty carpet; the body is that way, too. It will suck up that not-so-good nutrition more quickly after a fast. If a person takes in healthy food after the fast, however, it gets into cells and creates a higher level of health than existed before the fast. After a fast, eat foods with naturally occurring enzymes to help bring energy into your system and to help with digestion. Plants convert solar energy into matter through the process of photosynthesis. The closer we eat to that natural process, the easier it is for our digestion, and the more we bring in the basics we need.

For a beginner, a fast should last for only one day, unless it's done under the guidance of a physician. A "healing fast" can last anywhere from three to five days. One problem with this type of fast is that it puts the body into what is called a healing crisis, which is a period when it feels like symptoms have been exacerbated. That's normal, because the body is purging toxins, but people get scared when it happens because they think they are getting worse. Really, they're not. They should just hang in there until the crisis is alleviated. Eating well after the fast will bring energy into the system again.

In a simple juice fast, always use fresh juice, made either in a blender or a juicer, or you can squeeze fruit by hand. Drink juice throughout the day, as well as water, and do some simple walking. Moving becomes very important, as it not only flushes out your system but helps your lymphatic system. Read, meditate, listen to music; do this for twenty-four hours, and as you're coming out of the fast, you should add fresh soup or lightly steamed vegetables. And then, the next day, add rice or pasta to the fresh veggies and fruit.

When the body detoxifies itself, it releases energy that was used to hold toxins in. When those toxins are eliminated during fasting, that internal energy is freed, and your internal life force is freed. Fasting can raise nutrition to the level of the emotional, the mental, and the spiritual.

A person who is trying to heal should also do other things, such as yoga and *tai chi*, which help move the life force throughout the body. Stretching muscles improves circulation, moves oxygen into the muscle tissues, and helps eliminate toxins and debris from the body. The blood is the tonifying substance of the body, so the more a person moves around, the more opportunity life force has to move through the body.

When you're seeking a nutritionist, you should look for someone who understands about life force, who knows that food is more than just calories. You should ask the nutritionist about his or her treatment philosophy.

By doing some reading, you will be able to ask educated questions to get a sense of whether the nutritionist is in harmony with your own philosophy. There are books that address the issue of eating for health. One is *Healing with Whole Foods*, by Paul Pitchford; another is *Conscious Eating*, by Gabriel Cousens [see Bibliography]. Before people can start to make changes, their minds have to see that change is possible. The mind creates habits that say we have to live a certain way. So by reading, the mind gets in the act, too, and realizes it is possible to make these changes.

One thing to consider is the nutritionist's philosophy on spiritual nutrition. Most nutritionists stay at the purely scientific level, teaching that the body needs so many carbohydrates, so many proteins, x-amount of vitamin C, etc., to heal. And these things are all helpful, up to a point. But when dealing with a body that has a lot of toxins and a weak life force, there are more factors to consider than simple nutrition. A lot of nutritionists don't recognize that food has a certain life force of its own. A fresh apple is alive, but applesauce that has been cooked to a mush does not have any life force. It has calories, it has sugar, but no life force. And what people with chronic illnesses need is food that has life force. When you feel tremendous fatigue, do you feel like running a mile? No. Because there is very little life force.

This all sounds really wonderful. But we run into our own food-related habits. Where you first begin to make a change is an individual choice, based on your own awareness. Some people may have already made the shift to a more natural, wholesome diet. But making such a change may not even be in the consciousness of other people. You, as an individual, make changes based on your priorities.

The other thing that sneaks in is our judgment of ourselves, which oftentimes prevents us from making the move to a healthier diet. You know you should have an apple, but you really want to eat some chocolate. Go ahead and eat that candy; eat with deep awareness and joy. Then take that awareness to the next level, which is how you feel afterward. Ask yourself, "Is that how I want to feel?" And sometimes you're going to say, "It doesn't matter today." Other times, you're going to say, "No, I don't want to feel that way today." Peace comes from learning how to bring joy and awareness into your life. If you have joy and awareness, you don't have judgment.

Have you ever heard the saying that it takes a certain type of cook to make a good soup with heart? This means that person has a deep love and awareness about nourishment. If we bring our awareness into our food preparation, we infuse that food with our love and joy. That food then tastes differently, and that food has a different quality to it. I encourage everyone to practice with a very simple food, to see what you notice about it as you prepare it, to think of it with deep awareness as something you're choosing to nourish yourself with.

Here are the basic rules of eating. Try to keep your meals on a regular schedule, but if you don't feel hungry at mealtime, then fast until the next meal. Eat slowly, because your mouth is the juicer for your body, and it begins the digestion process. Eat only about four or five different kinds of food at one meal, because complexity makes digestion difficult. Don't snack between meals, and don't overload your system in one meal.

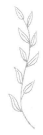

Eat until you're only half or three-quarters full. That should make you feel as if you've not really eaten. If you don't feel too full after eating, you've eaten the right meal. Maintain a peaceful attitude during meals, because if you infuse your meal with energy, your body experiences it on a higher level. Try to fast once a week or once every couple of weeks. Eat at least one raw salad a day, and try to shift from heavily cooked foods to lightly steamed foods. Always remember that you're eating to live, not living to eat.

A Patient's Story: Erin P.

Erin is thirty-three years old. She is an acupuncture student and is in a happy long-term relationship. She lives in Seattle, Washington.

Fear is what finally got me in to see the doctor. I had symptoms I had never heard of before, and I had no idea what was going on. The symptoms started in October 1992, very suddenly. I experienced tremendous amounts of pain and bleeding with my menstrual period, and a lot of fatigue, sleep problems, and pain in my neck, shoulders, and legs. I also had a lot of digestive disturbance, memory problems, concentration problems, and skin problems. I had to be careful about how much energy I expended, because I didn't have a lot in reserve. I visited three doctors before the fourth one finally diagnosed me with FM.

I have a history of urinary-tract infections, and I've taken a lot of antibiotics for them. In childhood, I had a lot of ear and upper-respiratory illnesses. I was born prematurely. I think I experienced food allergies, too, as a child. I also have had a lot of stress in my life, and a lot of grieving. My father had to leave when I was about fourteen to work in another state, and I lost him emotionally. Later on, in college, I had an intense relationship with a man, but we eventually broke up, and that was devastating for me.

Diet makes a dramatic difference for me. I went for a three-week detoxification program at a clinic in San Diego. They offer all kinds of treatments. I went mainly to do a cleanse, and I was just blown away by it. I was a little nervous when we first drove up. I thought, "Oh boy, what am I doing?" But it's very nice, it's simple, it's clean. They have a hot tub. They have a big dining room and an all-purpose room. It's sort of like going to camp; that's the way I think about it. We met a lot of really nice, interesting people there.

The cornerstone of the program is an all-raw-foods vegan diet, which sounds kind of boring, but I've been doing it at home and it's great. I have a lot of sprouts, and no animal products of any kind. Wheat-grass juice is a big part of it, too. Other parts of the program include colon cleansing, since the colon is phenomenally important in all bodily functions. If you have a lot of gunk built up in your intestines—which most of us do, due to our lifestyles—it permeates your whole body and clogs up everything. They taught us how to do a specific kind of daily lymphatic exercise—the lymphatic system is another waste disposal system in the body that can clog up. It's very easy to do and consists of leg lifts, stretches, and walking. It's very low impact, and it gets your lymphatic system moving. They also taught us ways to cultivate a positive mental attitude. The program cost $400 a week, which included room, board, classes, wheat grass, everything.

A lot of people go for one week, just to do a simple cleanse. By the time most people get through the first week, they feel a lot better. I felt terrible at first. I experienced all my FM symptoms about three times worse than usual during the first week. It wasn't easy. But my body was going through the detoxification process. All that stuff was coming out of my core and bubbling to the surface, and I was re-experiencing it both mentally and physically while it was being eliminated from my body.

By the middle of the second week, I started feeling a lot better. I ran up the same stairs that I had had a hard time walking down just two days before. I slept a lot better. My face started to look different. My boyfriend and I would both look in the mirror and go, "Oh, my God!" There was light emanating from my face; it was really a pretty sight. I felt a lot lighter and more unclogged. I felt clean inside, and it was easier to move, easier to think, because things weren't gunking up my system. It was really surprising.

The complete program runs for three weeks, and I'm really glad I was able to stay for the third week. It really tied things together. You go to classes the whole time you're there, and you learn about how your body works, how the foods you eat affect your body. Not only are you doing the cleansing process, you're also learning about why it's good for you, which really helps. I met another woman there who had FM. She was only able to stay for a week, and she still felt bad by the time she left.

I was amazed by the difference afterward. I didn't have any expectations about it, but I was able to sleep better than I ever have in my life.

I closed in a lot on myself when I got sick; I stopped socializing with people; I couldn't deal with people. I had to make huge lifestyle changes: leaving the corporate structure behind forever, changing the way I think about my body, the way I think about health. I'm now going back to school, partially as a result of having to learn all this stuff. I'm learning Chinese medicine. I'm really excited about it. I'm spending all my time doing this anyway, so I want to figure out how to make money doing it! My life is now nothing like it was when I first got sick. I'm a lot calmer and much more focused. When you're running on such a deficiency of mental acuity, you really have to focus to be able to do anything.

At first, it was embarrassing for me to be diagnosed with FM, because there's no societal acceptance of it. There's no allowance for people to be ill in our society, unless you have something really obvious, like cancer. I felt like I got a lot of disbelief from people. But a lot of positives have come out of this, even though it's been brutal. I think it's gotten me closer to where I want to be. You have to spend so much time going internally, because you've got no energy to be external. I had to sit with myself. At the time, I couldn't do much of anything else.

I would say that I am now 95 percent pain free. When I do experience pain, I do *chi kung* or some kind of exercise. When I need to, I go to the chiropractor, but that is very rare. I still haven't mastered the head fog, though. But I honestly believe that if I stick with this diet long enough, I will be completely well.

Naturopathy

Dr. Rebecca Wynsome

Naturopathic physician Dr. Rebecca Wynsome is consulted by physicians throughout the country for her expertise in using and interpreting the Female Hormone Panel, which is considered the most advanced lab test available for detecting and analyzing a woman's hormonal patterns. Her approach has produced dramatic benefits for patients suffering from hormonal problems, chronic problems related to allergies, and dysfunctions of the immune and digestive systems, all without the use of synthetic hormones or drugs.[1]

I am especially interested in natural hormone balancing and restoring body balance. I use several progressive, cutting-edge tests and therapies that can help people's body systems return to a more functional level. I consider myself a bridge builder, so I consult and coordinate with other health practitioners that my patients choose to consult. I work with patients and then refer them to acupuncturists, rheumatologists, internists, gastroenterologists, and other doctors when the need arises. I am not strictly "natural cure," as some naturopathic physicians are, which means they take all synthetic medications away from patients. I practice "functional medicine," which assesses how the body is actually doing and optimizes its functions. I practice health care, as opposed to disease care, which is more common in this country.

I'm involved with research on natural hormone use. Hormonal balance is important for people with FM and CFS (which are often related), most notably the adrenal hormones and the female, thyroid, and gut hormones; it's important to balance these in order to correct

---

[1] A portion of the information contained in this article was excerpted from Dr. Wynsome's publications *Your Comprehensive Health Rebuilding Program, More About Your Care in Our Clinic,* and *How Lab Tests Can Help.*

underlying imbalances that are in play in these syndromes. We perform a number of tests to check these hormones, and we use the outcome of these tests to help determine our course of treatment.

I help people with FM and CFS by first performing a thorough diagnostic work-up. I look specifically at the Adrenal Stress Index panel, because adrenal hormones have a powerful influence on energy, reproductive health, sleep, muscle and joint function, bone health, and the immune system. Because of our stressful lifestyles, poor diet, and other factors, the adrenal hormones are frequently out of balance. The Adrenal Stress Index test, which is a simple saliva test, determines how much cortisol and DHEA a person has. We also perform a thorough blood panel to check for such problems as anemia, organ dysfunction, immune system dysfunction, and nutrient deficiencies; we also check cholesterol, blood sugar, and blood type. I also test the stomach environment to find out if particles are passing unfiltered and unregulated into the system, thereby depositing byproducts in joint and muscle tissues.

I do these tests in context, though, using several other tests to determine what's going on for a patient. Once we know the root causes, then we use a rebuilding approach to achieve a stronger foundation within the patient's body.

My Health Rebuilding Program assesses and treats imbalances in the body's systems, using natural approaches that restore the body's ability to regulate itself. The Health Rebuilding Program is a structure that supports patients as they get well. I developed it, along with a corresponding notebook for patient use, through eight years of clinical practice, and its three phases have been adapted over the years to support patients in seeing their health in a new way. The Health Rebuilding Program is education-oriented, starting with the very first visit; we teach patients how to be in touch with their bodies. Each person's experience is different. Among the thousands of patients I have treated, no two were the same. I prepare an individualized plan for each patient, then reassess to see how their body is doing and to fine-tune the next step in their health recovery.

In Phase I, which we refer to as the "Relief" phase, we provide relief from discomfort, pain, malfunction, and lack of energy while simultaneously laying the foundation for complete recovery of the patient's health. A crucial component of this phase is metabolic clearing, which helps the body to dispose of accumulated waste products and helps heal the gastrointestinal tract. This is accomplished with a four-week, physician-supervised, modified nutritional diet program. Our convenient, healthy, nonfasting detoxification program gives every cell in the body a chance to resume optimal function. After this process, a person's organ systems are "up-regulated," so his or her liver works more effectively and the intestinal environment is much cleaner, which leads to less distress in the muscle and joint areas and also improves energy levels. The relief phase may also include physical therapy, if indicated by the patient's condition.

To avoid unnecessary complexity and to maintain a focus on getting results from metabolic clearing, specific nutrient therapy (supplements) are usually initiated in Phase II, the "Rebuilding" phase. Our priority now is to return the patient to a state of optimal health. Rebuilding health is like building a home. To have a home that is comfortable and functional, you ask an experienced, qualified architect to develop the plans. Then you implement the plans by laying a solid foundation. This is what we want to do with health.

The amount of time needed for rebuilding depends upon the seriousness of the patient's condition, and the rebuilding phase can take considerably longer than the relief phase. A treatment program during this phase may include hormone balancing, targeted nutrient therapy, organ function improvement, healthy lifestyle counseling, allergy desensitization, physical therapy, special detoxification programs, and in-depth laboratory assessment as needed.

I also use a supplement called Fibroplex, which has magnesium, malic acid, and several other nutrients to help restore normal body function. I prescribe DHEA when it's needed, and I also help lower cortisol levels through the use of amino acids, which help to correct chronic fatigue situations.

In Phase III, the "Maintenance" phase, our final goal is to help the patient maintain the state of optimal health that has been achieved through hard work and dedication. We don't want the patient to lose

135

ground and slip back into a state of ill health. Therefore, we provide patients with a program that will help keep them permanently free from disease and disability.

The health rebuilding process is a naturally evolving one. Patients who allow us to coach them have the best success. Many have commented that it has been worth their investment of time, energy, and finances. Many new patients, after their first visit, have said to me, "This is just what I was looking for." Others have said, "You asked me things about myself that have never been asked by a doctor before. I think you will be able to help me put my health puzzle pieces together."

It does require a leap of faith, at first, as this is a different kind of medical office than patients have ever been in before—different even than other naturopathic offices. Helping them to make this shift takes some astute listening and coaching on my part, especially in their first visit, and it takes some openness on their part. This is why I have developed the Health Rebuilding notebook, so that patients will have a resource to refer to and a record of the progress they make. We also show an introductory video to new patients to describe the working relationship we need to establish with them to ensure the best outcome for their health. We give them what we call the "patient success book," which shares other patients' success stories. These references help put legs under the patients' new beliefs about their health and recovery.

◼ A Patient's Story: David A.

David A. is a thirty-four-year-old who was a program manager at Microsoft when he became ill with FM. He and his wife currently reside in Seattle, Washington.

Working at Microsoft was one long trauma. There's a fair amount of stress involved, working twelve to fourteen hours a day and doing lots of computer work. No other disease would have had as great an impact on my life as the first moment that I realized I couldn't use my hands.

The pain in my wrists, upper arms, and shoulders was eventually diagnosed as carpal tunnel syndrome. I tried alternative treatments like chiropractic, massage therapy, and acupuncture, but I ended up having surgery on both wrists. I knew immediately that the surgery had failed: it helped my wrists for a few months, but it never addressed the pain in my arms or shoulders.

My illness developed over a period of time, and I just struggled through each new disabling condition. During that time I had my first migraine, and I started getting cravings for sugar. I was also much stiffer. I did yoga daily in an effort to loosen up. I also had much less tolerance for sitting down for long periods. My attention span decreased, too. I left work in February 1995 and went traveling for four months, but I got sick in the last month with some kind of intestinal thing. Within a few days of getting sick, I couldn't even walk. I had to cut my trip short. That triggered a whole host of new symptoms— pain in both feet, mental problems like spaciness, inability to concentrate, and irritability, and intensified food cravings.

I went to a doctor who suggested that I might have FM, but he did the trigger-point test and I wasn't sensitive in those areas, as far as I could tell. Later, I did find a doctor who diagnosed me with FM.

I typically turn to alternative medicine before I try Western medicine. In an effort to feel better, I decided to try the candida diet. I noticed a dramatic change. As soon as I cut out sugar, my mental acuity improved. The irritability went away; my concentration improved. That was the first clue that diet had a huge impact on my health.

It's critical that I stick to a regular diet. That means eating meals at the same time every day, eating similar kinds of foods, and eating certain quantities of food. If I don't eat enough, I get lightheaded and weak. If I eat too much, I overwhelm my digestive system. And I watch what I eat, of course. No wheat, no dairy, no sugar. I try to eat a lot of protein with every meal. I eat tuna, eggs, chicken, or tofu with lunch and dinner. I limit grains. My carbohydrates are mostly rice and a lot of steamed or stir-fried vegetables. Restaurant food can aggravate me.

It seems like a lot of people ignore diet. It's a change they're just not willing to make. They'll try everything else but won't change their diet. They either get a lot of pleasure out of their current diet or don't see the direct correlation between their diet and their health.

Being ill has forced me to do an elimination diet, and it's proven that I have to monitor my food intake. I tried vitamins for about six months, but I was spending sixty dollars a month on supplements alone and I didn't notice any huge change, other than that most of them seemed to end up in the toilet.

My life has definitely changed a lot since I got sick. I used to go backpacking or cross-country skiing every weekend or every other weekend. I met my wife while backpacking on Mt. Rainier. A big part of our relationship involved the outdoors, but we don't do that much now. I worked for Microsoft as a programmer, but now I can't even type anymore. I was a musician, a drummer, and I can't do that anymore, either. Those are the main compromises I've made.

I was very strongly linked to my physical activities, mentally and physically; they represented who I was as a person. I've had to totally redefine that and place less emphasis on my physical abilities. That's really changed my perspective on people, too. My ambitions—wanting to do it all, have it all, and be very active outdoors—have shrunk. It's hard to deal with sometimes. One of the hardest lessons to learn is that I am not my body.

Chapter 9

Exercise and Physical Therapy

T HE IMPORTANCE OF EXERCISE cannot be emphasized enough. In this chapter, you will hear from patients who regained strength and ease of movement through regular exercise and physical therapy. Although strenuous exercise should be avoided, you can benefit from low-impact exercise as long as it is consistently performed. Even fifteen minutes a day can make a significant impact on your mobility. Of course, you should check with your physician before beginning any new exercise regimen. To avoid flare-ups, start slowly, with a few minutes every other day, and work your way up to a longer exercise session.

Physical therapy is equally important, but it should be undertaken only with a licensed professional. If you don't already have a physical therapist, your doctor should be able to recommend one for you. The long-term benefits of physical therapy and exercise far outweigh the discomfort you may feel when you first begin your program.

For the person with FM or CFS, exercise isn't an option; it's a necessity. Dr. Robyn DeSautel, a chiropractor who practices in Seattle, is a proponent of regular exercise. "Exercising and stretching the muscles of the body will cause a reduction of symptoms in both CFS and FM," she says. "Many patients mistakenly believe that since they don't feel like moving, they shouldn't. However, motion is life. Lack of motion and resting too often create deterioration and lack of blood flow to the muscles, organs, and tissues. Increased blood flow through both cardiovascular exercise (which increases the heart rate) and stretching will strengthen the heart muscle, remove built-up toxins at the cellular level, and increase endorphins (the natural feel-good chemicals of the body). Exercise is most beneficial if done in short periods, twenty to thirty minutes, and repeated daily. It is repetition and consistency that cause permanent improvements.

"I suggest finding some activity that is enjoyable, convenient, and stimulating mentally and physically," she adds. "Daily activities such as dancing, yoga, brisk walking, or swimming will bring a better sense of mind/body connection and balance to patients challenged with FM or CFS."

The concept of physical therapy was developed after World War I to help treat injured soldiers, according to physical therapist and professor Dr. Kim Bennett. At that time, it was regarded as a rehabilitation science. "When the polio epidemic hit the United States in the 1940s and 1950s, it blossomed as a field," she says. "At that point, the focus was on musculoskeletal and neurological problems. We tried to help people who had been severely physically handicapped, either by their injuries or illnesses, to function as normally as possible. We learned that things like heat, electricity, and ice could calm muscles down and make people feel better. Massage, bracing, and splinting were all used to support joints that no longer functioned because nerves were dead or muscles were gone. Prosthetics came about because people had missing limbs due to war injuries.

"Now, we've begun to focus more on the traumas of our civilized society, including car accidents, overwork and stress, and weekend athletes who do too much and injure themselves. We also see patients who have traumatic spinal injuries and disc problems. We try to help them regain strength and to move correctly so that they don't reinjure themselves. There are many other areas of physical therapy; all are aimed at trying to maximize the physical potential a person has, to avoid abnormal movement patterns, and to make them as functional as possible."

Eduardo Barrera, a movement instructor, is someone who has benefited from a regular exercise program. He says he wandered through life with chronic fatigue, sleep problems, and pain in his back, hips, neck, shoulders, knees, and feet. Whatever activities he pursued, his coordination and endurance were poor. He would blow out some muscles, take some time to recover, and continue to try to play soccer. He took up mountain biking because his intuition told him that motion was good, even though it hurt like crazy. But his active life began to diminish. He had to do something about the continuing pain, so he tried massage, chiropractors, family doctors, osteopathic physicians, "Brain Gym" instructors, craniosacral therapists, physical therapy, postural reconstruction, massage, Hellerwork, Rolfing, meditation, *chi kung*, shiatsu, and acupuncture. He went on and off medications; he tried stretching exercises, reiki, *tai chi*, and yoga. Relief was temporary at best, and he became, in his words, "a difficult person to deal with." No therapy gave him anywhere near the success he has had with the exercise program known as Muscle Balance and Function Development.

Mari has been in the program since October 1998. One of the first things she noticed, after just a few short weeks, was the feeling of having both feet on the floor, her weight equally distributed between them. Also, she began to develop actual muscle tone and definition. "I kept making everyone feel my biceps because it was just so amazing!" Mari says. She felt her strength returning, and she wasn't injuring herself as much as she had before. "I did this program not so much to change the physical appearance of my body, but to get my body stronger so that I could lift things around the house and not constantly reinjure my back." Regular walking, too, has helped Mari in several ways: it's a good cardiovascular exercise, it's fun to do, and it's good to be out in the neighborhood. Mari says it's very peaceful and good for her mental health. She's decided that her feet can hurt just as much walking as they do while she's sitting and watching TV.

Physical therapy, as well as Muscle Balance and Function Development, has allowed Mari to hold her chiropractic adjustments longer, and the exercises she's learned in both modalities have helped her chronic back problems. She's been going to physical therapy off and on for years. The therapist she has been seeing most recently has done her the most good, because that therapist has taken time to diagnose which symptoms are related to FM and which are biomechanical.

A range of exercise options exists: physical therapy, yoga, *tai chi*, *chi kung*, and movement therapies such as the Alexander Technique [see Glossary]. Andrea recently began doing Tae-Bo, a combination of *tai chi* and boxing, and after just a few sessions she has experienced relaxation of a hamstring muscle that had been in constant spasm for four months. "I was doing a stretch and I just felt it ease back into place," Andrea says. She also reports a visible change in her body structure, although she hasn't even begun the regular workout session yet. "I'm going to keep at it as much as I can because I don't want to be using a walker when I'm sixty," she says.

Most of the people we've interviewed for this book agree that exercise and physical therapy have made a dramatic difference in their health. Tom O. says exercise is essential to his well being. "I am a firm believer in exercise. In the morning, I stretch, then I do push-ups, leg lifts, and other exercises to stretch myself out. It takes me twenty or twenty-five minutes. I just lie on the floor and roll over, back and forth, moving every little thing I can think of. That helps me a lot. Once I'm stretched out, I'm pretty much okay. I used to go walking for forty or fifty minutes every day on a trail near my house that goes straight uphill. I hurt my back, so I'm not able to do that anymore. But I still try to walk on a flat trail every day. And my work is active, too, so I don't sit all day."

Some people say they miss the active lifestyles they enjoyed before FM and CFS. Dennis H. says, "I used to play a lot of basketball, slow-pitch softball in the spring and summer, coed volleyball, water-skiing, tennis, and jogging. I didn't have other hobbies; I just took the sport of the season and did it. I enjoyed being physical, getting a lot of exercise. I'm not able to do all those activities now. I have no energy, and my body is all stiff muscles and joints. I go out walking in the evenings when I've had a temporary remission of my symptoms; those are my best times. I can break into a jog and not have my muscles and joints hurt."

Dennis reminds us that acceptance is the key to achieving some peace of mind for the chronically ill person. "I think you have to not compare yourself with what you used to do, or else you'll just drive yourself crazy, because the frustration level will be overwhelming. You shouldn't constantly remember or compare where you are now with where you were then."

Ann A. says that physical therapy helps. "It's gentle and careful therapy," she says. Ann also tried *tai chi*. "It worked well for a while, but then it seemed to not be beneficial anymore. I found, over the course of the last three or four years, that something will work for a while and then it won't. So I'll try something different. Right now, I'm doing yoga, and it's been very beneficial. The relaxation and stretching parts of it have been great."

For David A., physical therapy and myofascial release therapy help a lot. The third component of his treatment is exercise. "I swim every day, or I try to," he says. "I started out swimming ten minutes or so, and now I'm up to about forty-five minutes. I actually feel completely healthy the moment I get out of the pool, but after about an hour, of course, a lot of my symptoms return. But long term, swimming really improves my circulation. I don't have to sit around with multiple layers of clothing on anymore. I don't get head rushes when I stand up and my blood pressure goes up. I've tried some other exercises, but swimming is the only one that doesn't cause significant pain the next day or a few days afterward."

Melinda N. says, "I think exercise is important for people with FM. My exercise is belly dance. I have a certain regimen I do every morning; I used to do crunches, because I want to have a trim stomach, but the back of my neck was always aggravated. I bought one of those abdominal-roller bars. Now I can do sit-ups and the machine supports

143

the back of my neck. And then I do some belly-dance stretches. I continue to perform at local restaurants every seven or eight weeks, and that keeps me practicing. It would be so easy not to perform, but I know that if I don't, I'll stop practicing."

■ ■ ■

In this chapter we hope to persuade you to be as active as you possibly can. We are sure that inactivity is just about the worst thing we can do to ourselves. It is imperative to keep moving, even when we just want to curl up in bed. It doesn't matter which particular activity you choose. Just look for therapists and teachers that know how to work with FM and CFS, since you don't want to receive treatments or do exercises that are too strenuous for you.

■ Movement Therapy

Eduardo Barrera

Eduardo Barrera is a Muscle Balance and Function Development therapist and operates the GravityWerks clinic in Seattle, Washington. He also has FM.

In 1997, an acupuncturist suggested that I start doing an exercise program from a book. Some of the stretches were familiar: gentle yoga postures and other motions such as squeezing a pillow between my knees. The next time the acupuncturist saw me, he noticed a change in my posture. My massage therapist noticed that I was loosening up too. In a relatively short time, my pains receded, and for the first time I felt both feet on the ground, literally. I had no idea about balance; it was a theoretical concept in my life. As I improved, however, the fog left, my vision cleared, the stiffness left. I knew I was venturing into new territory.

I was so thrilled. I knew I had to get involved in movement ther-

144

apy. My clinic, understandably, would not train me, so I ventured to learn it on my own, which proved to be a sophomoric attempt until more good luck came along. A small article in a magazine mentioned a program called Muscle Balance and Function Development (MBF). This led me to Geoff Gluckman, the former assistant director of a San Diego clinic, who now teaches the science behind his program all over the world.

MBF is a systematic, scientifically based exercise/motion program that looks at a person's compensations within the three cardinal planes of movement—in other words, the three primary ranges of movement. When you walk, with your arms and legs moving, that is one range. The second range is moving your arms and legs out to the sides, doing jumping jacks, for example. The third range is rotating or twisting your body. The intersection of these three planes is roughly your center of gravity—that is, if you are in alignment. Each time you move, this center changes. If there are any interruptions or misalignments, your entire structure is compromised.

This program brings your body back into postural realignment through a series of sequential exercises that retrain the neuromuscular system. These movement exercises remind the muscles of their original function.

Proper alignment allows the body to move with ease and efficiency. Our bodies have to contend with gravity, and that's much easier if the main weight-bearing joints are vertically aligned and horizontally parallel with each other and with the ground—the shoulders over the hips, hips over the knees, knees over the ankles, with the feet pointing straight ahead. Each side of the body bears half the weight, which is known as proper load bearing. The muscles and tendons are less likely to be strained and restricted. Proper alignment also allows internal organs to function properly. Less energy and effort are required if the body exhibits true alignment.

Those who live with FM, CFS, or chronic pain nearly always exhibit unsatisfactory balance and increased fatigue. Along with that, they usually have poor posture. (This posture is identified in the book *Muscles Testing and Function,* by Florence Peterson Kendall, Elizabeth

Kendall McCreary, and Patricia Geise Provance; see Bibliography.) If we were to drop a string from the ceiling to the floor, it would represent the line of gravity. The major weight-bearing joints are vertically aligned with this line. But most people with FM exhibit a posture that is not functionally aligned in relation to gravity. Those with CFS are in the same boat, but their bodies show more of a rotational posture around the line of gravity. People with FM usually display a posture with the head, shoulder joints, and hip joints forward (a sort of "ski-jumper" position). People with CFS usually have a hip or shoulder that rotates farther forward than its counterpart. People with both FM and CFS display aberrant postures depending on their illness; this may explain some of the similar symptoms.

Fatigued bodies use more energy than necessary because they constantly fight the gravitational line. Each day becomes an athletic event as you try to remain upright. Some muscles overreact, and the others go along for the ride. Even though your muscles are in a state of imbalance, however, your body compensates and allows you to "live with it." This causes a lack of flexibility, and pain is caused by persistent misalignment. The longer your history of imbalance, the greater your propensity for pain. Compensations, misalignment, and absence of proper neurological signals due to faulty load bearing reduce the body's ability to exercise or perform activities of daily life. This leads people to decrease their activity, which increases muscular atrophy and causes further compensations. In other words, there is a cycle, and this may be why pain seems to move around and surface in different areas at different times. It is this underlying compensation cycle that needs to be addressed.

When scientists at NASA studied weightlessness and gravity, they used bed rest to reproduce zero gravity. Recall how the astronauts appear after a space mission, all rubbery-legged from not using their muscles in relation to earth's gravity. Their studies proved the devastating effects of inactivity and lack of motion on the body. Within twenty-four to seventy-two hours of inactivity, the muscular system begins to break down. In some people, it takes a mere eight hours, an average workday if you are desk-bound. The cycle of inactivity is perpetuated in our daily lives and our muscles lose their functional capacity without us even noticing. And if one engages in repetitive activities without proper alignment, that will cause compensations; thus, no matter how healthy the activity, the pain will not diminish.

Especially for the chronically ill person, overexercising can be as harmful as getting no exercise at all. An article in the August 1998 issue of the *Penn State Sports Medicine Newsletter* reported symptoms of exercise overtraining: depression, anxiety, sleep disorders, swollen lymph nodes, irregularity in bowel function, upper-respiratory infections, and unusual soreness. Sound familiar? Bet you didn't know that you were an overtrained athlete!

The body is sending the message that it wants to move, it needs to move, it has to move; it just needs a little help getting back on its proper path. I kept moving all the years of my illness, but I didn't have the right foundation and I kept "crashing" afterward. This condition can be corrected by restoring the proper neurological pathways to the body through a systematic reeducation of muscle function. The MBF technique applies principles of physics and biomechanics to help restore postural realignment.

The MBF method is unique, since it actually restores functionality to the body. It allows me to live a life that is a complete reversal of my former life. I feel well almost every day, and I have never felt this well in my life. It's as if night has been turned into day and I can participate in life more than ever before. Those sports I used to play in pain are now played without pain and with pleasure.

The following four sequential MBF exercises can help to promote balance for some individuals. First, lie down on your back in front of a chair and rest your feet and lower legs on the chair cushion or seat. Your arms may lie at your sides, palms facing up, or you may rest your hands on your stomach. In other words, you are creating right angles in your legs, at ninety degrees, in relation to your body. Lie there and breathe from your diaphragm. Place a piece of paper on your stomach and move it up and down with each breath. Lie there for five to ten minutes, letting your hips, back, and shoulders fall into the floor.

Next, lie on your back and place your feet flat on the floor with your knees bent, arms at your side. Place a soccer ball or pillow between your knees and begin your breathing while pressing the knees evenly together and then releasing without dropping the ball. Do this twenty times. Ideally, you could do this exercise in three sets of twenty, although it is not necessary to begin at that level. Ask yourself where you feel this exercise working.

Then remove the ball and remain in the same position, hands by your sides, palms up, and gently squeeze your shoulder blades together and release them. Try this twenty times at first and work up to three sets of twenty. As you do this motion, you should be able to feel both sides of your shoulders working. They may be doing different things, and that's okay.

The fourth exercise will tie in all the work you have done. Find a wall against which you can lean. Place your back against the wall and slide down it into a ninety-degree position. Align your feet so they are pointing straight and are in line with your knees and hips. If you can't get down that far, that's okay; just lower yourself to a comfortable place. Check to make sure your ankles are not behind your knees. You want to establish a right angle. Then press the small of your back into the wall while relaxing your stomach, and breathe. Try to hold this position for two minutes. If your legs tremble, that's okay, too. You are reintroducing functional strength into your thighs. If the position becomes unbearable, raise yourself higher and continue breathing.

Through these exercises, you are reintroducing functional movement and providing yourself with neuromuscular reeducation. Over time, you will increase your ability through repetition. With practice and by increasing the number of repetitions, the body will remember how to do it.

MBF is an individual process, since everyone has his or her own unique compensations that need to be rebalanced. The purpose is to reestablish the body's balance and function in reference to the force of gravity and return the body to its maximum level of function. You can do this yourself, without any special equipment, devices, or manipulations. It is a most natural way of health care. To regain control of your physical well-being and the feeling of flexibility and balance, all you need is yourself. You can provide yourself with the foundation for effortless movement and balance.

The MBF program works within a person's present level of ability. As the body changes, other motions are introduced to help reinforce proper structure. It has allowed me to walk, bend, reach, climb, do as I please, once my body returned to a more functional state. I feel better, I live pain free, and I do not have to be dependent on medication my whole life.

If you are in pain, please know that you don't have to "live with it." I am living proof that this program works. It has been the missing link in my lifestyle. It is part of my daily hygiene, my foundation for movement. My life is now filled with days of wellness, joy, and happiness. Others have achieved this, too; in fact, my former acupuncturist and *tai chi* instructor are now my clients.

A Patient's Story: Sherry J.

Sherry, fifty-eight, lives in Tacoma, Washington, with her husband. They have three adult children. She has both FM and CFS, and has participated in Muscle Balance and Function Development training.

I was diagnosed with FM at least twenty years ago, early on, when it was still called "fibrocitis." I had a brand-new young doctor right out of medical school, and she had a friend who was a rheumatologist. It was one of those coincidental things: because they were both so young, they knew something about it. She didn't know how to treat it, but she referred me to the rheumatologist and he diagnosed the fibrocitis. He gave me a lot of helpful hints; a lot of them kept me on my feet.

About eight years ago, I was slipping so fast it was unreal. I began to lose cognition; I couldn't make change anymore; I would show up late for my own art shows. I caught a bad virus, too. I spent three or four weeks with a high fever. I think that kicked off the CFS, because

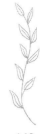

149

I never came back to full capacity after that.

Just recently, I've started a movement therapy program called Muscle Balance and Function Development that stresses total body alignment and mindful breathing as a way to strengthen the body. I now have less pain and more strength in my body as a result of doing these exercises. I started slowly and built to an hour a day, and it's really changed how I feel. Before I started the program, I never made any morning appointments, period. It had to be almost life or death. I'd sleep till noon every day. But now, after religiously following the movement program, I'm awake at 9:30 A.M. every day, and I take much less pain medication than I did before.

Exercise has made a world of difference in my life. I have a full routine of physical therapy exercises I do, along with movement exercises every night before I go to bed. If I stop exercising, within a week and a half my right knee would collapse and I would probably fall somewhere, so I have to keep doing it.

My FM and CFS are getting worse as I get older. But I'm better off now, because I have learned how to manage my illness and because I exercise. To any new diagnosed person, I would emphatically say this—you have to have an exercise program. No matter how badly you feel, no matter if you think you can't do it, your body will deteriorate if you don't do it. You will lose ground if you do not exercise!

Physical Therapy

Dr. Kim Bennett

Dr. Kim Bennett works with a group of physical therapists in private practice at Olympic Physical Therapy in Seattle. She also teaches gross anatomy and is a clinical assistant professor of rehabilitation medicine at the University of Washington. She wrote two chapters on therapeutic exercise for *Therapeutic Exercise: Moving Toward Function,* edited by C. Hall and L. Thein-Brody [see Bibliography].

I'm very interested in people. I love to know about people's backgrounds, their lives and all of that. That's probably one of the things that helps me to treat FM patients, because so many factors affect FM, and because it in turn has an effect on so many parts of my patients' lives. It helps to have a full picture. The more I understand about the lives of the people I treat, the better job I'm able to do. Since I started physical therapy, I've become interested in people who have multiple problems that are typically chronic in nature. Rarely do my patients come in with just a sprained ankle. Usually, it's something that's been going on for a long time, and many parts of their body may be involved.

How can physical therapy help FM and CFS sufferers? One of the interventions for people with FM is exercise—but, as anyone with FM knows, exercise is a double-edged sword. If you do it right, it can be helpful. But it is easy to do it wrong, to overexert and have it set you back. Part of my role as a physical therapist is to help people learn how to progress their exercise and to convince them that holding back is really better than "just doing it."

Another way that physical therapy benefits FM and CFS patients is through hands-on work to treat areas of pain. I see a lot of FM and CFS patients who are sedentary, or perhaps do not always rest in good postures, so they push themselves out of alignment. I frequently see people with headaches, shoulder problems, or low-back pain; this generalized pain has gotten lumped in as part of the FM or CFS diagnosis. But in reality, it is a problem that a person without FM/CFS might have, too, just because their body is in poor alignment or perhaps because they have a hypermobile system that has been in poor alignment too long. I treat biomechanical problems in which joints aren't lining up correctly and are causing pain and movement problems. Much of my treatment is aimed at addressing specific physical faults that really have a sound biomechanical reason for existing.

For example, I might work on a shoulder joint that is out of alignment and perhaps eliminate the discomfort that causes a person to awaken in the middle of the night. If we can eliminate that problem, it's a step toward getting the patient to sleep better.

There are some common patterns in CFS/FM patients that I find very interesting. It's common that people with FM are very intelligent high achievers, but they might also be hypervigilant worriers, responsible for everybody, never quite letting themselves rest. They're constantly in a state of anxiety, worrying about what's coming next. It has been argued that there's a high incidence of either verbal or physical abuse in the backgrounds of people with FM and CFS. That, too, may play into this hypervigilance—people in chronic pain are watching out to avoid an attack all the time.

I believe that stress and imbalance in the autonomic nervous system—the part that causes either the fight-or-flight response (the sympathetic) or relaxation (the parasympathetic)—can cause some of the symptoms commonly seen in FM and CFS patients. The sympathetic part gets way too active, and the parasympathetic part isn't active enough. Physical therapy teaches relaxation techniques and other tricks to increase the activity of the parasympathetic system and to decrease sympathetic activity.

To achieve these treatment goals, I teach people progressive relaxation (a type of meditation), biofeedback techniques, and proper breathing. People with FM tend to hold their breath or be upper-chest breathers, which is an abnormal breathing pattern that can contribute to pain as well as result from it. Another really important part of physical therapy is teaching people to treat themselves and to make better use of resources. Most of the people with FM whom I've met are highly informed about available resources, but occasionally I'll meet someone who is newly diagnosed or has not reached out into the community to see what's available around them. So part of my responsibility is to get them to read books or look up other resources. For example, there are massage and acupuncture schools that will provide their services for a low payment or sometimes for no payment at all.

As part of patient education, we also talk a lot about pacing—not just in exercise, but in everyday life. I teach my patients how to treat themselves using ice, heat, and electrical stimulation. Almost everything that I do to people to get their joints back in alignment, I can teach them to do to themselves with some degree of efficiency. We try to get people to realize that there are a lot of different tools; we try to find the thing that will work for the individual patient.

Your physical therapist should specialize in treating people with FM or CFS. If I had either condition and I didn't know who to go to, I would ask my physician who they send their patients to, so that I'd know I was going to somebody with experience. If you don't have that option, I would strongly recommend calling therapists directly and asking them to explain what they do. There are therapists who are so busy that they wouldn't have time to do that, and I think you would want to avoid those people in general. If their priority is not patient education, you probably don't want to see them either. Once you are in treatment, if you have concerns about how things are going, discuss them to be sure you are on the same wavelength as your therapist.

If you can't find someone who has experience specifically with these conditions, the next best step is talking to a physical therapist who has experience working with one of the rheumatoid diseases, like rheumatoid arthritis, or another chronic condition in which the therapist needs to be gentle. A number of orthopedic physical therapists deal primarily with sports injuries, and their expectations about levels of performance may be too intense for people with FM or CFS. No matter which provider you see, however, be prepared to be told that some level of exercise is essential to healing.

I do not like to recommend exercise without first having seen someone. It's a very individual process. But probably very gentle stretching exercises are okay. I think that the book called *Stretching*, by Bob Anderson and Jean E. Anderson, is sound [see Bibliography]. People with FM or CFS should use their fatigue or their pain as a limit, because sometimes they won't know for twenty-four hours if what they're doing is too much. If you start an exercise program, start with one or two exercises on the first day, do them for only a minute or two, but no more, and see how you feel twenty-four hours later. If you're okay, then you might add one more exercise.

This is the area in which I experience the most challenge with my patients, especially if they have worked out in the past. You have to reframe your attitude toward exercise. Instead of patting yourself on

153

the back because you've just run two miles, you have to pat yourself on the back because you've held back and only run for two minutes this time. Your reward is for your discipline in holding back, rather than for your discipline in going out and exercising. It takes people with FM or CFS longer to work into an exercise program that is really helpful.

The Arthritis Foundation offers a lot of exercise classes for people with arthritis, and I have been involved in training people who teach those courses. I know that they are reliable, and they follow strict guidelines, because they are set up to protect the rheumatoid arthritis patient [see Resources]. Their water aerobics may help, especially because you do these exercises underwater, and this helps to reduce gravity. These exercises are very slow in their progression. The Foundation insists that the pools in which the aerobics are taught must be at least eighty-nine degrees, with only a small difference in the air temperature, so it can't be too cold outside the pool. The pools have to be accessible, easily gotten into and out of. That's one less stress for somebody who has FM or CFS.

As far as other exercises go, try walking. For some people, walking half a mile will be fine. For others, walking from the front door to the mailbox and back is a challenge. Sometimes people need to do more limited walking, but they should try to do it every day. And it has to be purposeless exercise, done for relaxation, as well. Hopefully it can be kind of mindless; people shouldn't just say, "Well, I've just parked the car and walked to the dry cleaners and back." I truly believe that exercise pulls you into a different part of your brain; it increases endorphins and gets you away from the physical world. And those are only a few benefits of exercise.

I recommend four books on the subject of coping with life [see Bibliography]. I love them because their authors are really down-to-earth, funny and wise and nonjudgmental, and when I read them I feel better. One of them is *Full Catastrophe Living*, by Jon Kabat-Zinn. It has an especially wonderful chapter on not overreacting to events. I think having that attitude about life is a great tool for somebody with FM or CFS. The other book is *Minding the Body, Mending the Mind*, by Joan Borysenko. She's one of the first people to write about the mind/body connection. She is a neuroimmunopsychocellular biologist, which means that she studies cell biology and immune reactions as they are involved in mind-driven events. She also has wonderful ideas for coping with life and taking care of yourself.

There is another self-help book with some great ideas. The author is Barbara Penner, and the book is *Managing Fibromyalgia: A Six-Week Course on Self-Care*. I use it for my patients; I give them handouts. Another book that's helpful is *Fibromyalgia Syndrome: Getting Healthy*, by Jeanne Melvin. The Arthritis Foundation also has many useful publications.

People with CFS and FM need to learn to live with their condition. They have some symptoms that are fixable; physical therapy can help with those. But more than that, physical therapy is an education process about how to live with a physical problem. It teaches you to use the tools of physical therapy to treat yourself. That's a good reason to go through the physical therapy process. When you participate in physical therapy, be sure you are allowed to be an equal team member in your treatment plan, and that you are treated as if you have the ultimate responsibility for taking care of your body. Be mindful of insurance restrictions, and be sure your visits are planned accordingly. After all, you are the consumer.

■ A Patient's Story: Betty M.

Betty M. is thirty-six years old and was a florist before she became ill. She's been in a relationship with her girlfriend for nine years. They live with their dogs and cats and fish in Seattle.

Over the last five years, I have met so many FM and CFS people who are reluctant to exercise because they believe it will aggravate their condition. I couldn't disagree more. Since I began my physical therapy and movement therapy exercises, I have found I have less morning stiffness and less pain when I'm sitting, and I have real muscle tone for the first time in years. I encourage people to find an exercise

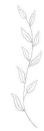

155

that is fun for them, so that they are more likely to do it on a regular basis. I exercise an average of six days a week. If I don't exercise, I feel worse when I wake up in the morning.

The stretching exercises I learned in my yoga class have helped the most. I try to stretch every day; this helps keep my back and leg muscles from getting so tight. I try to walk a few blocks in my neighborhood every day. That has been most helpful for my depression—just getting out and moving around outside has been beneficial.

Years of constant pain in my feet and legs led me to find a solution. In April 1988, my right foot began to hurt suddenly, just a whisper of pain on top of the foot and around the ankle. By the end of the day, the pain was not a whisper but a shout. The doctor thought I'd sprained it, but by the next week the pain was in both feet. By then, it was screaming at me!

I was a florist at the time, and it wasn't uncommon for me to work fifteen hours a day during a holiday week. I loved my job as a designer in a big shop downtown. I thrived on the fast pace and stress of the holidays: ordering flowers, rushing to fill orders, interacting with busy customers. My favorite part of the day was when I would first arrive at work in the morning and turn on the lights. There would be a whole cooler full of bright flowers and a scent like no other. Words cannot describe how great it was to be around beautiful, colorful flowers all day, creating bouquets and making my customers happy.

But it became harder and harder for me to stand all day. I designed arrangements while sitting as much as possible, but I missed the rhythm and speed of my "old" feet because designing arrangements is like a dance. Eventually, I left my downtown job for a management position at a smaller neighborhood shop. I began to work fewer hours and relied more on my coworkers for help.

For years, I went from doctor to podiatrist and back again trying to find out what was wrong with my feet. I tried injections, anti-inflammatories, heat, cold, physical therapy, you name it. Nothing seemed to help but rest, and I couldn't rest much because I had to work. Then came the diagnosis: tarsal tunnel syndrome. In 1991, the "cure" for this was a release operation similar to the one done for carpal tunnel syndrome in the hands. I decided to go for it. I thought my feet couldn't possibly hurt as much after the surgery as they did now. I had the operation, and within one month I was back to work. What a mistake! As soon as I resumed my old work habits, the pain returned. In fact, having my feet cut open didn't hurt as much as the tarsal tunnel pain. And over the next year, I developed pain all over my body, along with bone-crushing fatigue.

Getting through work became more and more intolerable, and my world began to get smaller and smaller as it shrunk to just work and rest, rest and work. My feet were now more painful than ever. On Christmas Eve 1994, after months of misery, pain, and indecision, I knew I had no choice but to leave my job for good. I remember sitting alone in the dark on my last day at work, after I had closed the shop and put everything away, thinking, "Well, this is it."

Before the holidays, I had concentrated on wrapping up my duties at work, hiring someone to do my job, training her, getting organized at home. Every few minutes, I would have to sit down and rest because the pain was so intense. If I had to stand for any length of time, in line at the grocery store, for example, I had to bounce from foot to foot. Like carpal tunnel, the more you use your feet, the more they hurt. I had such a hard time with my feet that I hadn't even had time to think about how I would feel when suddenly, after thirteen years, I didn't have a job to go to.

Surprisingly, it was my podiatrist who thought I might have FM. Four months after I gave up my job, I was diagnosed with FM and shortly thereafter with CFS. A real turning point for me was when I met my physical therapist. She's a great diagnostician; she was the only physical therapist who took the time to really work with me. She was the only doctor who was able to figure out which symptoms were FM-related and which were related to biomechanical problems. She figured out the source of the pain in my legs and gave me exercises to stretch and strengthen my muscles. She taught me exercises that I do at home every day to try to combat a rib that pops out of place. I've realized that myofascial release actually works and that hands-on treatment, like massage, actually helps me. I can also have ultrasound

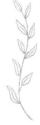

and other therapies besides just exercise when I go for an office visit. Physical therapy has made a big difference in my back problems. When I first went to see my therapist, I was unable to even sit comfortably. Now my posture has changed and my back is so much better because of our work together! Doing my physical therapy exercises on a regular basis keeps me limber enough so I don't constantly reinjure myself.

Another piece of the treatment puzzle fell into place when I met my new podiatrist. He fashioned orthotics for me that helped decrease the pain in my feet for the first time in ten years. Although my tarsal tunnel condition will probably never completely heal, I can now squeeze my feet across their widest part and not feel any pain at all. I've been able to stand and walk for longer periods without having to take constant breaks.

Through my rheumatologist, I found treatment for FM. Through the Arthritis Foundation, I found a support group. My support group has been invaluable in helping me adjust to living with a chronic pain condition. I encourage everyone with FM and/or CFS to contact the Arthritis Foundation for a list of support groups in their area [see Resources]. I once thought that my doctors would be the ones who fixed me, and that I would be just a casual observer in that process. But I began to understand that I was a partner with my care providers in my own healing. The more I took charge of my care plan, the more personal power I received in return.

Once I knew what medications to take for my illness, I looked for alternative treatments that I could do in conjunction with my Western medicine approach. Many treatments give me relief: craniosacral manipulation, acupuncture, and energetic healing. Today I include chiropractic adjustments on a weekly basis, which greatly reduce the intensity of my almost-daily headaches. I also take Levoxyl for my Hashimoto's disease, which is a common thyroid condition. Visualization and meditation help me cope with the pain.

I only see people and do things when I'm feeling well. (To get to that point, though, I must use narcotic pain medications.) Nobody ever sees me when I'm feeling badly, because I tend to stay at home with my pets and rest as much as I can. People don't understand that

I'm in pain, because they only see me when I'm smiling and laughing. I make every effort to be a happy person, and I'm not going to change my personality just to fit somebody else's misconception of what a sick person should look like.

Right now, there is no cure for FM or CFS, but it is up to me to find ways to live with it as best I can. Exercise is a big part of that philosophy. My biggest challenge has been finding a balance between getting enough rest and feeling like I'm a part of things. At this point, my energy level is about 20 percent of what it used to be. The pain itself is a daily challenge. But I've learned to not give up pleasure just because my energy is too limited to allow me to do the activities I used to enjoy. New things give me pleasure, like watching my cats play, reading, and watching movies. I divide my tasks into manageable parts, and rest in between them. I nap and meditate. I try to remain positive and optimistic. The realization that my FM pain is cyclical helps me to know that I will not feel this bad every day of my life. As long as I exercise at least six days a week, I feel like I can exercise some measure of control over my life.

Yoga

Vijay Elarth

Vijay Elarth is a certified yoga instructor and owner of the Karuna Integral Yoga Center in Seattle. Vijay has practiced yoga since 1979. He became certified to teach integral yoga in 1984, and in 1985 he became certified to teach advanced classes.

Yoga is an Eastern exercise and movement therapy designed to restore harmony, flexibility, and function to the body. I didn't begin yoga until I was in my mid-forties. It made me feel so good that I wanted to do more with my body than just sit around and watch television. People tend to think yoga is only stretching, but part of the yoga practice works with organs and other systems of the body. I also like the ben-

159

efits of the deep relaxation when the body is quiet; then the energies of the body flow into the immune system, and all of this helps keep the body active.

I try to teach very gentle movements, and after we move for a short while, we rest in what's called a restorative pose. It's the resting poses, when the body does no work or very little work, that allow the body to be renewed. This, combined with gentle stretching and deep relaxation, strengthens the body's immune system. Hopefully, this can benefit people who have FM or CFS. Particularly for them, the important thing is to bring movement to the body without increasing the level of pain.

Cleansing poses are among the most beneficial for people with FM or CFS. In the forward bend, we squeeze the liver and stretch the kidneys, which helps them do their job better. These organs help the body cleanse itself, so anything that benefits them also helps the body to be more efficient in its work.

Janusirshasana, often translated as "head-to-knee pose," is one of the best cleansing poses. For this pose, sit on the floor with the right leg straight and the left knee bent, pressing the sole of the left foot against the inside of the right leg wherever comfortable. Then fold from the hips over the right thigh. As the abdomen comes closer to the thigh, the liver is squeezed and the kidneys are stretched. Beginners should hold this pose for perhaps fifteen seconds, then repeat. Those more experienced in the pose will be able to hold it for up to one minute. After folding over the right thigh, reverse the legs and fold over the left thigh.

There is a caution about this pose, though. People with lower-back problems will increase tensions during the forward bend unless they move into the pose correctly and very slowly. To avoid building tension in the lower back, inhale deeply to extend the spine upward before folding over either thigh. Then, holding the breath and the extension, fold until the body reaches its limit of comfort, and then exhale. At this point, the head can be relaxed so that it drifts toward the knee. Sometimes after this pose, people say they have a slightly bitter but not unpleasant taste in their mouths. I believe that this is the result of the liver's being stimulated to do its job well. After this pose, I usually offer a sip of water.

Another cleansing practice is *uddhiyana bandha*, the stomach lift. For this pose, stand with the feet about shoulder width apart, then exhale completely and lean forward. The knees are slightly bent. Place the hands on the knees, then raise the head. Lift the abdomen in and up, hold it until you feel like you need to inhale, then release the abdomen and stand, and inhale gently. It is beneficial to repeat this three times, and to do so while the stomach is empty of food. Caution: This cleansing practice may increase the flow of blood during menstruation; it is best to avoid it at that time. This practice is said to help prevent or cure digestive problems, especially constipation.

Much pain is caused by poor posture. An important pose for strengthening the spinal erector muscles is *arddha salabasana*, the half-locust pose. Lie on the abdomen with the legs straight and together. Place the hands, palm up, under the thighs or hips. Then stretch the right leg and lift it slightly into the air. The knees should be kept straight. The right foot can be held in any comfortable position. Beginners can hold this pose for perhaps fifteen seconds, rest for a moment, then repeat. As the body strengthens, the pose can be held for up to one minute. Repeat the pose, raising the left leg. During the pose, as during most poses, avoid the temptation to hold your breath. Let it do as it wishes.

I believe breathing practices are of great benefit to those with CFS or FM because they help to release toxins and impurities from the body. The basic breathing practice is *deergha swasam*, the three-part breath. This can be done while sitting in a chair with the spine straight but not stiff. Take control of the breath, then exhale deeply from the abdomen. Let the inhalation begin in the abdomen, flow through the lower chest, then rise into the upper chest. When it reaches the upper chest, the collarbones may slightly rise. Then exhale from the collarbones, deep into the abdomen. This is one breath. In the beginning, continue the practice for a couple of minutes, gradually lengthening the time up to five minutes.

In my opinion, a yoga teacher should have three qualities. A yoga teacher should be certified. The yoga teacher should be a student of some other teacher, preferably of a different tradition of yoga. (There are many traditions of yoga; some are very gentle, which is what I teach, and others are very strenuous. The yoga teacher should have experience with all these traditions.) Finally, the yoga teacher should have basic knowledge of the structures of the body and how the systems of the body work. The yoga teacher should be able to name the muscles. If you ask a teacher where the biceps are, and he or she says, "In the legs," go elsewhere. They should also be able to name the bones of the skeleton.

Several books offer more information about yoga poses and cleansing practices: *Integral Yoga Hatha*, by Swami Satchidananda; *The Sivananda Companion to Yoga*, by the Sivananda Yoga Center; and *Yoga of the Heart*, by Jenny Beeken [see Bibliography].

Most yoga is pretty strenuous. And whether a person with FM or CFS can find a class that's gentle and mild, like my classes, I can't say. But if you look for the word "Integral" in class names, these teachers should be of the tradition of gentle and quiet yoga practice. Integral is the key.

◾ A Patient's Story: Rebecca H.

Rebecca is a forty-eight-year-old lesbian and has lived in Seattle for twenty-two years. Her advice to chronically ill people is simple: keep moving. She wishes good luck and good health to us all.

Like many people with FM, I have a long history of physical and emotional trauma. I grew up in an abusive home. My father was abusive. I had surgery when I was just nine hours old because I was born with my liver extruding. When I was seven, I jumped off a two-story building. We were being daredevils. It didn't do my body much good.

When I first found out I had FM, part of me felt happy to have a name for what was bothering me. It just reinforced what I already knew, but I didn't feel too good about it because I knew FM is serious. I used to work in factories before I came out to Seattle and became a welder. I worked in the shipyards and other places, and the fact that I could do it meant that I could take care of myself financially. Now I can't do that work anymore because my hands and shoulders are shot. And I can't say, "Oh, I'll just go and pull espresso if I have to."

I started going to *chi kung* two years ago. My doctor actually recommended it, because I was falling all the time. I fell seven times in six months, hurting my body all over again with each fall. We talked about how many times I had fallen, and she said, "You need to get your balance back in the world." So I went to a special-health-needs *chi kung* class. It combines mindful breathing and movement. It's gentle and easy on the body. At first, I needed to sit down in class for a good twenty minutes and then stand the rest of the time, which is kind of difficult for me, but I did it anyway. Before long, we were outside in the summertime in the park, and I realized I was standing the whole hour and it was okay. It totally and tremendously relaxed my body. It was so incredible to go in there and do the class and feel no pain in my body, to just be totally relaxed by the end of the class. It was wonderful. When you have FM and your body hurts all the time, it's hard to imagine a day when it doesn't hurt.

The *chi kung* class turned into a *tai chi* class. It was kind of frustrating, because I couldn't remember all the forms at first. Nobody does. But once I learned my forms, it felt good and I started doing home practice. I became addicted to it, because it felt so good and I was so relaxed. I had to do it three times a day, every day. It strengthens your body; it improves blood circulation and bone density. It helps you relax and get stronger.

I have an on-and-off fear of the future now. I don't feel like I have as many work options as I had before, because of my illness. I feel real limited. I can do different things, but it's tough. It's scary to lose part of your independence. I try to find things to replace what I've lost, but I have to set limits. If I do work in the yard, I do it in fifteen-minute increments. I try to stay positive. I do all the things I have to do to take care of myself, much more than I did before I became ill. Lately, I've been working heavily with my spirituality, focusing on the

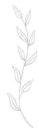

body and spirit connection. Part of me is ill, and that does affect me emotionally and spiritually. When you don't feel well or your body hurts, you can't be who you know you are in your own body.

I try to do a lot of reading, listening to tapes; I do my exercises, work on healing the mind and the body, and work on acceptance. I'm forgiving a lot of events that happened to me in my childhood, I mean really forgiving and letting them go. Things I've hung onto from the past may be causing my blockages now, so I'm working on them. I want to heal. I want to be better some day. I have it in my head that I'm going to be healthy again, and I don't know if that's denial. Some people believe if you have FM, then you have it forever. But I'm going to leave myself the option of being well.

Chapter 10

Other
Healing Options

THIS CHAPTER OUTLINES additional treatment possibilities that the person with FM or CFS should explore. Often, people turn to these options after they have exhausted more traditional therapies. Many times, though, it is a combination of therapies that provides the best results. Anyone who has a chronic, painful condition that can't be satisfactorily treated or managed with more traditional approaches may want to get involved with such options as naturopathy, homeopathy, or Chinese medicine, which are discussed elsewhere in this book. People may also wish to try more unusual approaches, like craniosacral therapy or oxygen therapy, which, while not necessarily "doctor approved," can be beneficial. These options are discussed in detail in this chapter.

Many physicians don't object to patients trying a range of different healing options; in fact, physicians often hear testimonials from their FM or CFS patients regarding improvement of pain and fatigue after trying these types of treatments. Despite the fact that little empirical data exist to shore up the claims that "alternative" treatments can provide a miracle cure, you should feel free to experiment with as many treatment options as possible, as long as they are not harmful and don't deplete your wallet too much. And remember that some treatments, unfortunately, may be scams, so be cautious in the treatment decisions you make.

Many years of hopeful trial and error led Mari and Andrea to seek relief from their own symptoms through numerous alternative therapies, including the following:

- orthotics

- energetic healing sessions provided by a spiritual healer

- yoga

- acupuncture

- reflexology (massage at pressure points on the hands and feet)

- massage therapy

- hot-tub therapy

- tennis balls (used in acupressure)

- osteopathic manipulation

- water aerobics

- chocolate therapy

- magnet therapy (the use of magnets on painful points on the body)

- positive visualization (creating visual imagery in the mind to bring about healing)

- meditation

- spiritual cleansing rituals

- colonic cleansings

In addition to trying these and other alternative therapies, we also radically changed our diets (see Chapter 8). But there's no magic pill—believe us, we would have found it after a combined eight years of searching for a cure.

The people we interviewed for this book also described a surprising range of alternative therapies. "Many of us have gone to extreme measures to try to alleviate our pain," said sixty-one-year-old Bea R. "I was so pleased to have even gotten a diagnosis from my doctor that if he said, 'Take a little arsenic every day,' I would have done it."

Ellen J. uses one of the more unconventional treatments for her FM and multiple chemical sensitivity. "One of my treatments is oxygen therapy. It's considered a drug. It was originally prescribed for my chemical sensitivity. My psychiatrist actually prescribed it because I kept being late to his office or wouldn't be able to make it all, because I'd get so lost trying to drive there. The therapy has really helped a lot with the cognitive difficulties. I am now able to drive without getting lost. But the side benefit was that my pain level decreased quite a bit, too.

"When I went to see my rheumatologist, I expected him to kind of pooh-pooh the idea, but he actually was very supportive. He's not prescribing it for everybody, but he gave me some research that showed that people with FM actually desaturate at night, which means that the level of oxygen their cells take in during the night is much lower than normal. The study found that the lack of oxygen reaching the tissues could be a big reason why FM people have so much pain. The longer I'm on it, the sharper I am. I use it when I leave the house now. I use it when I'm driving and when I go into stores and doctors' offices, which are notoriously bad places to breathe the air.

"Since I have multiple chemical sensitivity," Ellen says, "my naturopath has also done a lot of nutrient therapy. I have a tube in my chest through which I can infuse vitamins and minerals. It has helped with the chemical sensitivity, and my migraines are now under control. My neurologist thinks that's because of the B vitamins. The migraines were being triggered by muscle tension from the FM. I used to have to go to the emergency room at least once a month, and I was in the neurologist's office several times a month to get pain injections. Also, I've been able to decrease and stabilize to a certain extent on some of my other pain medications. At least my level of pain hasn't gone up; though there are times where I have significant pain, I have been able to manage them because of the nutritional therapy."

Other people have found relief with a microcurrent unit, which delivers an electrical impulse that interrupts pain messages to the brain. The device is palm-sized, runs on a nine-volt battery, and has two wires that attach to electrodes. These wires deliver a low-level electrical current to the patient. Nancy Campbell distributes the Alpha Stim 100, a microcurrent unit [see Resources]. "These units can be helpful for people with FM and sometimes CFS," she says. "They're useful for more things than pain relief, too. Physical therapists use them to deliver electrical current around an injured area to induce the site to heal."

The unit may be used in three different ways:

- Use the electrodes. If you've had a TENS unit (another type of device used to send electrical impulses through a patient's body), then you know what the electrodes are—patches that you put on your body, and the wires deliver the current to them. The electrodes have a sticky gel on them, and they can be reused. The electrodes are used when you're going to leave the unit on for long periods of time. Treatment is most effective when all four electrodes are crossed through the pain site.

- Use the probes. The probes attach to the wires and are used instead of electrodes. They are good for FM patients because the probes enable the patient to "chase" the pain.

- Use the ear clips for cranial-electric simulation (CES). Ear clips are little cotton pads that, when moistened and clipped onto the ears, deliver a very low-level current through the brain. CES is also useful for anxiety, insomnia, and depression.

"Microcurrent units are especially good for headaches," Nancy says. "They work for any kind of facial pain, including TMJ pain. It's important to not wait until the headache spikes, until the pain gets really bad. I think women do that a lot, thinking that we can push through it. When you start feeling a headache coming on, that's when you start using the ear clips. If the clips don't get rid of the pain, use the probes, one on either temple. There's no need to put them on your eyes. As you get the probes close to the eyes, you may see flashing lights if you close your eyes, but that's okay. There are two things that you need to remember when you're working with electrical current. One: Use at least two electrodes, so that the current has a place to go. Two: You must use saline solution or water to moisten the pads.

"The microcurrent unit is not the answer to everyone's problems," Nancy says, "but it is an especially useful tool for the FM patient to have." Strangely, what works for one person completely bombs for another. Mari experienced a lot of relief using the Alpha Stim, while Andrea is a little leery of attaching herself to electrodes.

Massage therapy, too, works for many people, but not for everyone: Andrea experienced excellent results with massage, while Mari did not. Fifty-two-year-old Sharon W., who has had FM for almost twenty-five years, has found out the hard way that getting regular massage is an irreplaceable part of her treatment regimen. "I started getting massages a number of years ago, and they felt so good that I just kept them up," she says. "I discovered it wasn't a luxury; it was something I needed to do on a regular basis to feel better. If I have a bad day, I still have golf-ball-sized knots on my muscles."

Perseverance can pay off. Some people actually do experience a remission-type relief from symptoms. Jody E. was so sick at one point that she questioned whether she would have to drop out of school. She was fortunate enough to find a doctor who prescribed a mouth orthotic, which supports jaw function and allows for easier breathing. Jody's treatment involved the use of this intraoral orthotic called a splint. The splint also has special patented extensions that allow the tongue to elevate out of the throat. Jody wore this appliance most of the time in the beginning, even though it held her jaw in an unusual position.

The first day she wore the appliance, Jody still had shoulder pain, but there was more mobility in her neck, her head posture was more erect, and she slept more than nine hours that night! Her doctor made an adjustment to the orthotic, and the residual shoulder pain dissolved within seconds. A week later, Jody reported increased energy. After treatment with orthotics, breath and posture training, and muscle strengthening, Jody's posture is nearly normal. Six weeks into her care, Jody says she is more active and sleeping well, and her fibromyalgia points are no longer painful. She has stopped taking medication altogether and is active and feeling well.

There are many other treatment options available that can help alleviate the symptoms of FM and CFS; it's just a matter of finding the ones that work for you. This chapter explains a few that we haven't described in detail elsewhere.

Craniosacral Therapy

Cherste Nilde

Cherste Nilde, L.M.T., is a licensed massage therapist who practices craniosacral release therapy (CSR, an osteopathic technique) in Kaneohe, Hawaii. She works with both FM and CFS patients. She says that while performing craniosacral work on a client, she often finds blocks in the system that are literally created by emotional or physical trauma. Those blocks can be released by craniosacral therapy, which can actually bring out traumatic memories—sometimes a specific physical movement or position echoes the one that the body was in when the injury occurred. CSR can help the client release stored-up energy.

When patients first come in for a craniosacral treatment, I have them lie down on the table. You can use different positions, depending on what the patient is comfortable with, but flat on the back is what I usually start out with. I generally start by checking all the body systems. One of the methods I use to find energy blocks in the body is called "manual thermal diagnosis." This is a scanning of the body's energy field; I follow the different hot or cold, "buzzy" or dead sensations at different levels of the patient's body, which I can literally feel through my hands.

During a craniosacral treatment, I can feel a restriction in movement when I manipulate the patient's cranial bones, scalp, and neck. This is how I know where a release needs to occur. I am tuning into restrictions in motion in the body. I let the body lead me to the barrier where motion stops and stored-up energy has been generated by the patient's body as a response to injury or stress. Craniosacral manipulation pushes through that block and enhances movement as well as the flow of healing energy throughout the system.

Some people are very attuned to physical movements and even energetic sensations in their systems, and they can feel all of the therapy that's happening to them. Other people cannot feel it at all, but it's still happening; some people simply have more awareness than others. When I use my hands to manipulate the cranial bones, it can sometimes feel very dramatic to the patient, like a lot of muscles are moving in one area, or like something is being stretched and expanded, although the patient can't really name what that "something" is. Sometimes it just feels like a membrane, a tissue, or ball of energy that's growing and spreading; even the bones can change in that area. Sometimes, it almost feels like a procedure such as angioplasty, in which a balloon is inserted into an injured area and expanded. Those sensations give me a pretty good idea of what I'm finding in certain areas of the patient's body and what areas of temperature difference in the body might be related to. There are different ways to discover problems in a patient. A lot of times, the body part that the person is complaining about is not where the problem actually is. Pain can be referred from another area—the block may be located elsewhere in the system.

I learned to perform craniosacral therapy from a teacher who studied at the Upledger Institute. Its base is in Florida, but its teachers travel all over the world to train practitioners. I also practice Somato-Emotional Release (SER), which is another similar cranial manipulation technique. We are finding that memories are stored not only in the brain, but also in the tissues, and these memories—such as memories of physical abuse, trauma, or illness—can be emotional as well as physical. SER can help heal those blocks by bringing them to the surface and freeing them so that the body can process them.

Healing can occur once these memories have been brought to the surface. The patient might not be aware of the full impact of an experience; for example, a person who has been in an auto accident may not have really dealt with all the fear and rage that were involved on top of the physical injuries. Those emotions have helped hold that injury in the patient's system rather than letting it heal. The places in the body where these emotions are trapped are called "energy cysts."

Cranial work is subtle enough that it doesn't create resistance in the tissues and allows the practitioner to work gently in the damaged areas. Tissues that are in chronic pain or are hypersensitive resist heavy-duty stretching or exercise if they haven't gradually built up to it. But because craniosacral therapy is a low-impact treatment that can also affect the body's neurological function, it seems to have the ability to calm a hypersensitized system, especially in the case of people with FM or CFS. The craniosacral practitioner can provide a greater range of motion and make a greater impact without the stress to the patient's system that strenuous exercise would cause.

Craniosacral treatment helps to free up movement throughout the whole body, not just in the affected area, and it helps to stimulate and reawaken the tissues. It helps with lymphatic drainage and circulation of spinal fluids. It also can help localize different injuries or focal points in the nervous system that other treatments can't affect. I work with people who have developed CFS or FM symptoms; they tie together in different areas that really affect the whole nervous system.

For the person who is interested in giving craniosacral therapy a try, calling the Upledger Institute in West Palm Beach, Florida [see Resources], would be a good way to find practitioners throughout the country. Or you could call around in your local area until you find someone who offers this type of therapy. You'll have to try it and see how that particular person works for you. The cost differs depending on what kind of practitioner you visit, but massage therapy generally costs less than physical therapy.

Craniosacral work is definitely getting more popular in recent years. People like Dr. Andrew Weil are helping to publicize it more, and more practitioners are now available than ever before. I became a proponent of craniosacral by receiving it myself—it was so dramatic for me that I knew I needed to learn how to do it myself. I view this therapy as one of the treatment choices that the practice of medicine will move toward, as it's much less invasive than surgery or pharmaceutical medicine.

■ A Patient's Story: Becky R.

Becky is thirty-two years old and lives with her partner in Seattle. They have three guinea pigs and one cat. She has tried a variety of techniques, including physical therapy, chiropractic, and naturopathy, to deal with the symptoms of her CFS. But, as she reminds us, there is no quick fix to the problems related to chronic illness.

When I became ill, I had just finished college and was kind of in transition. In 1989, I developed a bad sinus infection; it was the first one I ever had. It hung on, and I have never shaken it since. What motivated me to finally go to the doctor was finding that I couldn't function. I was diagnosed fairly quickly. I was really lucky I found my current doctor, because I had heard horror stories from other people about bad doctors.

I had a major trauma in college; the guy I was dating was killed in a freak accident. When my CFS was diagnosed, I didn't draw any connection with that at all. But recently, I've heard people talk about the fact that trauma can trigger CFS and FM in some people. I don't know if that really triggered it, but it probably had something to do with it.

I think I have all the symptoms of CFS: the chronic sore throat and sinus problems, and a bit of depression. I've done physical therapy for my neck; I've done acupuncture for neck pain and chronic

173

fatigue; I've done chiropractic; I've done it all, with temporary relief. The neck pain, especially, seems to come and go in these vicious cycles: if my neck hurts, it keeps me up at night and then the fatigue is very bad. When the fatigue is bad, I kind of lie around, which makes my neck worse. I feel like there's some inherent weakness in my body and it's manifesting itself in all these different ways. It's never been confirmed that my symptoms are related.

Some days it gets bad, but most of the time, it's maybe a two or three on a scale of one to ten. At least I can function. It goes up occasionally, when I go into cycles and the fatigue tends to get worse.

They have a physical medicine department at my clinic, so I'm seeing a naturopath for fatigue and digestive issues, and I get a lot of massage treatment and craniosacral work. The clinic is right around the corner from my home, which is great. Seeing the naturopathic doctors has really opened my eyes to the fact that the body is a system. It amazes me, the power the body can have—if there's one little thing out of whack, it influences the entire system. This differs from the view of conventional doctors, who try to treat each individual symptom. I've learned to look at my body as my own.

My new naturopath began treating the chronic neck pain and was more effective than any providers I had seen previously. When I began complaining more and more about my constant sluggishness, fatigue, and weight gain, and the fact that they seemed to be getting worse despite the antidepressant medication I was taking, she began talking about a thyroid condition called Wilson's Syndrome.

I mentioned that I had previously had several blood tests to screen for hypothyroidism, and all were within "normal limits," even though my symptoms seemed to be consistent with an underactive thyroid. My naturopath explained to me that thyroid tests measure the amount of inactive thyroid hormone in the body. Wilson's Syndrome is a condition in which the body is not able to convert inactive hormone into active usable hormone. So a blood test could be normal and there still could be hypothyroid conditions occurring. To confirm this possible diagnosis, she asked me to check my basal body temperature every day for two weeks. Sure enough, my temperature was consistently in a range significantly lower than 98.6 degrees Fahrenheit. I began taking liothyronine (T3 hormone).

This condition seems similar to CFS/FM but this is not recognized by many doctors as anything more than unproven rhetoric. Yet after only a few days on T3, my basal body temperature rose to a normal level, and it stabilized after three weeks on the medication. I was able to finally quit taking antidepressant medication, and I do not miss it at all! My naturopath also validated my hunch that my neck pain might be related to the fatigue and depression. I have noticed that my worst days, energy-wise, are also the ones when my neck hurts the most.

We are continuing to treat my neck pain with physical therapy, exercises, and chiropractic adjustments. My energy level over the last few weeks has been higher than I can remember in many years. And I feel like the "fog" is finally beginning to lift. I strongly encourage anyone who is dealing with chronic fatigue, pain, or depression to explore Wilson's Syndrome as a possibility. The national Wilson's Syndrome Foundation has a Web site [see Resources].

I'm learning to discipline myself better as far as my eating habits are concerned. There are still some days when I just have to have some Ben & Jerry's, but I've learned to make it an occasional treat instead of a staple. And I've learned that when I'm knocked-down-dragged-out tired, I need to accept it and forget whatever else I had planned to do, because if I'm that tired, I need to rest. I've missed a lot of things I wanted to do because I've been too tired, but I'm learning to not plan so much. What I really need to do is rest.

In the long run, my life has changed for the better, because I've become so much more aware of my pain. I learned a technique in which I spent an hour or so every day blocking out the external and turning my senses inside. It was something that actually brought quite a bit of pleasure into my life. But I found I was too tired to do it on a daily basis. That's what made me say, "Enough is enough." I can deal with taking a day off work here and there, but when I wasn't even up to fulfilling my own contentment every day, I knew that something drastic had to happen.

In the spring of 1990, I met my spiritual teacher. That's been an incredible journey, and it continues in self-awareness and self-appreciation. I don't think you can call it work on a spiritual level, because it's a lot more tangible, but on a practical level I've really been working on being aware of my illness. My situation hasn't changed, but working on my spiritual health has given me more energy to deal with my illness. You can't get better until you accept it.

■ Massage Therapy

Noreen Flack

Noreen Flack is a licensed massage practitioner at the Seattle Acupuncture Associates clinic, where she has worked for five years. Noreen graduated from the Brian Utting School of Massage in 1993 and is a member of the American Massage Therapy Association. Massage is gaining more acceptance as an adjunct therapy for people with FM and CFS.

Our practitioners offer alternative approaches for people who suffer from chronic pain and who haven't had a lot of success with Western medicine. We see a lot of patients who suffer from different types of illnesses and diseases and haven't found a lot of relief with their current treatment plans. They come to the center to try "new" things, like acupuncture, massage therapy, physical therapy, counseling, biofeedback, and occupational therapy. Although these patients are trying alternative treatment, they might not necessarily be open to it because they haven't had much success with anything else; they're just willing to experiment further.

Typically, a person will first fill out an intake form. I ask several questions to get an idea of what results they are expecting, what they're there for, and what medications they're on, so I can have an idea of where they're at in their treatment, whether there are any known side effects of their medications, and how their medications might affect their muscle tissues. Then we go back to the massage room. I like to keep it on the warm side, so the patient can relax easily. The lighting is low, there's a bit of aromatherapy in the air, and the music is soft and relaxing. The therapy environment is very important, so that the patient can feel comfortable and relax their mind as well as their body. Then I find out what their goals and expectations are, so I can have an idea of how to treat them specifically. I specialize in many different massage techniques and therapies, so I can adjust my treatment depending on the type of person and the result they're looking for.

For example, if someone comes in with a whiplash or muscle strain or sprain, I would probably work locally at the site of injury to try to draw out any scar tissue or adhesions from the injury, which would decrease inflammation and help heal that area. I would also try to relax them so that their healing response can increase. If someone comes in with depression, I might do a full-body massage that's very relaxing, very light, to help them let go of any stress they're carrying so their muscles can relax and dilate.

I think an FM patient should go to a massage therapist who has experience with treating that specific type of illness, rather than just going in for a massage and receiving the same treatment the therapist might give to someone who just wants to relax.

With a CFS or FM patient, I usually listen to their story first. A lot of times there's a huge emotional component that I try to address, because they have been suffering not only physical pain but emotional pain. They're oftentimes frustrated; they've seen very few results by the time they come to me; they're discouraged and even depressed. I can empathize with their plight, because they are experiencing a sympathetic response to the stressful situation that they're in. Their muscles are constricted, their breathing is usually shallow, and they're very "bound up" in their bodies. There are a lot of holding patterns; there's a lot of guarding.

It's really interesting to work with people with FM. It's also challenging, because there is no set groundwork and your skills have to be very diverse to be able to help everyone. Even with the same FM patient, you wouldn't necessarily do the same treatment every time.

Someone with a muscle strain or sprain would be treated the same way every time.

The first session is critical in assessing the person, getting a feel for where they're at with their illness. If a person has been recently diagnosed, I would probably be very cautious and conservative in their treatment. I usually treat people with FM or CFS very lightly in the beginning. A lot of times, people who have just been diagnosed with FM are feeling pain in certain points of their bodies, and they want me to specifically address those points; people want me to really dig deep into those painful areas. But addressing those specific points isn't necessarily going to do them a lot of good; that can actually cause a much more severe flare-up the next day, so I have to explain to them how massage affects them. During the session, it feels good, but that's not necessarily true in the case of a person with FM. I think it's dangerous, because it can be so painful the next day that you've actually done a lot more harm than good.

In order to start working with patients, you have to create a safe place to get them to calm down, feel safe, and feel like someone is trying to help them, that someone has empathy for them. I try to make a connection with patients on an emotional level without doing any actual counseling. I think many of my patients also see mental-health counselors and are trying to deal with their emotional issues. A safe environment, especially in the first few sessions, is vital, so that the patient can decide whether they like you, if they like being touched by you. Chances are that they're going to relax more and they're going to have a better healing response in a safe and comfortable environment than if they feel uncomfortable and the practitioner is just digging away into their rigid muscle tissues.

I normally use something like craniosacral therapy, which is very gentle, and a lot of times the patient doesn't feel anything because I'm just holding my hand on pressure points. But, in fact, when they get up off the table, they recognize that something good has happened. Usually, a huge part of that feeling comes from their own commitment to healing; it's not necessarily anything the therapist has done. A lot of what I do is just give them the opportunity to get grounded for themselves and go inward—their own healing response has actually addressed the points that they've been complaining about, rather than resisting. When you get into a cycle of resistance, it's so much harder to get anywhere; it's like bumping heads rather than going with the flow.

Massage has so many benefits for people with FM; it's just incredible. If you have had a bad experience with massage therapy, I encourage you to go to someone who has experience in treating this particular problem. Massage can be very beneficial when done correctly, but it can also be very painful if you go to the wrong person. If you can find a therapist who is experienced in this syndrome, I think you'll feel much better.

Massage is good, but you shouldn't expect to be cured by massage. In conjunction with other therapies, it can be very beneficial; it will help you feel better faster and allow you to make more progress because it helps to stimulate something within yourself. It can get you on the road to recovery a lot faster and help you feel better on a day-to-day basis.

Chapter 11

The Narcotics Controversy

SOMETIMES IT CAN TAKE YEARS before a patient finally admits that narcotics are the next step in their treatment plan. We don't want to be addicted, we don't want the additional expense or side effects, and we don't want the social stigma attached to narcotic consumption. Many of us exhaust all other possibilities before finally deciding to give narcotics a try. Making that painful decision, however, is just the beginning of the battle. Narcotics are a valid treatment option, but obtaining them can be complicated at best.

In this chapter, we hope to defuse some of the volatility of this subject. You will learn about the variety of medications available, as well as hear a cautionary tale or two about what unanticipated roadblocks may lie along the way. We hope the newly diagnosed person will not be scared away from this treatment option by others' ignorance, arrogance, or misinformation.

A major problem that FM and CFS patients have to contend with during the healing process is the hesitation of physicians to prescribe narcotics because they fear reprimand from medical boards and suspension of their license to practice medicine. Research shows that only 12 percent of physicians surveyed are willing to prescribe narcotics for people with nonmalignant pain. Another problem is the misconception that narcotics do not work on FM or CFS pain. Compounding these problems are physicians who will not prescribe narcotics for fear that the patient will become addicted. Finally, there's the misconception that once we begin taking opioids, we will need increasingly higher dosages to get the same pain relief. Mari says she went through a lot of trial and error to find a narcotic pain medication she could tolerate, but when she finally did find Oxycodone, she was able to take the same dosage for several years and wasn't dependent on an ever-increasing dose.

For the people fortunate enough to obtain a prescription for narcotics, taking the drug may be the only thing that's helped them function. Andrew M. says, "I finally found a doctor who is willing to help me with some pain medication, and it has changed my life. It's taken the edge off so that FM doesn't have to be the dominating force in my life all day, every day. I had a hard time getting a doctor to help me with this, and I have been working a long time to get this kind of help. I take ten milligrams of methadone three times a day. Most people don't think of methadone for pain relief, but it works well for me. The doctor wanted to put me on some expensive time-released narcotic drug called Oxycontin, but that's not generic, and for thirty tablets they want a hundred dollars. And if it can't be gotten generically, I have to pay half. My doctor's second choice was the methadone, which is working well. I told him I didn't expect to be pain free. I just wanted something to help.

"The first thing he told me when I asked for pain medication— remember, this is supposed to be a pain management specialist—is that opiates don't work well for people with FM. And I said I knew an FM patient who was getting pain medication and it worked for her. My doctor said, 'There's always the exception,' and prescribed it. It's

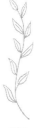

181

made my life worth living again. It's made all the difference."

Other patients have been able to find pain relief only through a combination of drugs. "I take Serzone, which is an antidepressant," says Sandra W. "I'm on Ambien, which is a sleeping medication, and I also take methadone. At first, I thought, 'They use methadone to take people off heroin, right? Now I'm going to take heroin.' Even though methadone is only a synthetic substitute they use to take people off heroin, I had a negative connotation going before I even tried it.

"But I started taking it, and it took about a week and a half for it to kick in. To wake up and not have pain in the morning, to not have to deal with that on a daily basis, was pretty amazing. It was very emotional for me. Before, I hated taking medication, and I hated the fact that my former husband would call me a drug addict, because he doesn't even take aspirin. So I had to deal with stigma, too—people making value judgments on what I was doing to my own body. The methadone has allowed me to function." As for people who would call her a drug addict, Sandra wants them to know this: "I don't get 'high' on methadone; I get hope."

Other patients have intentionally become outlaws because they use medical marijuana to treat their pain. These people are either exceptionally desperate, brave, or foolhardy, since any person who uses marijuana (even for medicinal purposes) runs the risk of incurring monetary fines, federal forfeiture, and mandatory minimum jail sentences. Marijuana is currently classified by the federal government as a Schedule I narcotic, which puts it in the same regulatory classification as heroin and LSD. Under federal law, doctors are not allowed to prescribe these substances under any circumstances. This does not stop people from giving it a try. Annie D. reports that she feels more relief from two puffs of pot than from a whole month's worth of expensive muscle relaxants. She is fortunate enough to live in one of the seven states with medical marijuana laws on the books. Millions of other people in this country risk their freedom to use this illegal medication.

Other countries, such as the Netherlands and England, have either legalized or decriminalized the use of "soft" drugs. Vancouver, British Columbia, resident Marc Emery is waging a one-man war against the law of the land in Canada. The publisher of the pro-marijuana magazine *Cannabis Culture*, he ran a business in Vancouver named Hemp B.C. At one time, this upscale head shop featured a grow room that offered technical information in addition to selling hemp clothing, oil, soap, and smoking accouterments. Marc finally sold the business last year, but he continues to sell seeds by mail and risks his freedom in the process. He was invited to visit the United States, but he said that wasn't likely to happen anytime soon. "They blame me for the increase in marijuana production in Canada and the U.S.," Marc says. "They may be right!"

This chapter is not designed to persuade you to break the law, but to help you make a more informed decision about the use of narcotics to help control your pain. As patients, we shouldn't have to live in pain every day if there are medications to help alleviate that suffering. It is worth your time to continue to interview doctors until you find one who is willing to prescribe these medications, if that's the decision you make.

Medical Treatment with Opiates

Dr. Michael Young

Dr. Michael Young served as medical director of an adolescent chemical dependency program from 1986 to 1987, as well as medical director of a 250-physician managed care organization. He is author of the book *Unbelievable Pain*.

I had my medical license restricted by the Washington State Medical Quality Assurance Commission (MQAC) between April 1997 and March 1998 for "overprescribing" narcotics to four patients with chronic nonmalignant pain. Naturally, doctors are wary of prescribing narcotics for long-term pain for several reasons: fear of causing addiction, fear of side effects (constipation, lethargy, respiratory depression), and lack of experience in treatment of chronic pain. A more pressing

fear is, of course, loss of licensing. Relevant to this fear are the attitudes of medical disciplinary boards. Jorensen et al. reported the following in the *Federal Bulletin* 1992 regarding medical board attitudes on narcotics prescription:

It is legal and legitimate to treat...	*% agreeing*
Cancer pain	75
Cancer pain with history of opioid abuse	46
Chronic nonmalignant pain	12
Chronic nonmalignant pain with history of opioid abuse	1

A majority of physician still believe that treatment of chronic nonmalignant pain with narcotics (i.e., opioid analgesics) is almost never appropriate, and practitioners who continue to prescribe this form of treatment are at risk of sanctions and restrictions from their medical board. The practical effect of any restriction, which is the minimum action taken by the board, is loss of one's ability to practice. Most physicians are not willing to risk losing their license for the sake of providing pain relief. Most, but not all.

Many doctors are also unwilling to risk a patient becoming addicted, although this risk is negligible in chronic-pain patients. We know now that addiction is largely biologically determined and that not everyone can become addicted. The number of people at risk in the general population for opiate addiction is unknown, but it is certainly below 10 percent. The dilemma of treatment can be illustrated by posing the following question: Assuming a 10 percent risk of addiction upon exposure to opiates for every ten people who present with chronic intractable pain that is unresponsive to treatment other than narcotic medications, and if one of these people will become addicted to the treatment, is it ethical to withhold treatment from the other nine to avoid the risk of addicting the one? I say the answer to that question is "No," and an emphatic "NO!" when you consider that the actual risk is far below 10 percent.

The use of marijuana for medicinal purposes is a current controversy and adds confusion to the treatment of chronic-pain conditions.

While the effects of marijuana are limited to euphoria, appetite stimulation, and relief of nausea, it may have benefit in pain treatment, but evidence for this is anecdotal. Furthermore, marijuana has a long regulatory history. Its prescriptive form, Marinol, is indicated for use as an antinausea agent and for appetite stimulation. Whether because of side effects, lack of effectiveness, or stigma, Marinol is rarely prescribed by the general practitioner. The undertreatment of pain is such a serious and pervasive issue, and the introduction of marijuana use only clouds the debate.

Narcotic analgesics such as Oxycodone, on the other hand, are a proven and effective treatment for chronic nonmalignant pain. I have cared for patients who have been incapacitated and unable to accomplish activities of daily life, much less hold down a job, due to chronic pain. These same patients have successfully returned to work and recovered joy in their life with safe doses of narcotics, suffering no adverse affects. They are able to maintain scheduled doses without tolerance or addiction. Ironically, risk of addiction in treatment of chronic pain is low. In a Boston collaborative drug study, only four out of 11,882 patients treated with opiates became addicted. In national burn centers, none of the 10,000 patients treated became addicted. Of 2,369 patients treated for migraine headaches, only three became addicted.

Surprisingly, narcotic analgesics sometimes have fewer side effects than some of the other therapies. Not everyone responds to these medications, however. Like everything else, narcotics should only be tried after patients have exhausted other options. A trial on narcotic analgesics is then reasonable for those people. Careful adherence to prescriptive guidelines is especially important with these medications.

In the treatment of FM with narcotics, however, I do have some reservations. First, I believe alternative therapies should be tried and exhausted. Second, I believe treatment of depression should be addressed as well. Finally, I believe a written contract for the proper and safe use of opioid drugs should be made and honored. With those caveats, I believe there is a place for treatment with narcotics for patients with FM.

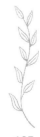

185

Other therapies to be considered in the treatment of FM include the following:

- tricyclic antidepressants or selective serotonin reuptake inhibitors (SSRIs) like Effexor, which can reduce pain; Trazodone is preferred to Elavil

- NSAIDs (nonsteroidal anti-inflammatory drugs)

- Tylenol

- Ultram (a pain medication that inhibits serotonin and norepinephrine reuptake—do not exceed 400 milligrams per day)

- magnesium

- DHEA (dehydroepiandrosterone, the most prevalent hormone in the human body)

- Robaxin, Flexeril, Soma, Skelaxin (muscle relaxants)

A multidisciplinary approach for treatment of FM includes the following:

- education

- counseling

- biofeedback

- sleep quality

- *tai chi*

- exercise

- physical therapy

- occupational therapy

- acupuncture

- cognitive and behavioral therapy

You will notice an absence of opiates in these lists, except for the inclusion of Ultram. Curiously, Ultram is a morphine-receptor agonist that produces tolerance and withdrawal, constipation, and seizures (similar to Demerol) and has been repeatedly abused. These features are common to almost all opiates, yet Ultram is still unscheduled and advertised as a "non-narcotic." Codeine is a much cheaper and safer substitute, yet it is controlled and scheduled and also puts the provider at risk for regulatory scrutiny.

■ A Patient's Story: Melinda N.

Melinda, fifty-two years old, is married. She has FM. She and her husband have two children, and the family lives in Seattle. She developed FM after a car accident.

For the first six months after the car accident, all I did was go to the doctor and cry. I feel like I lost about three years of my life. Before I got hurt, I used to just jump out of bed. My husband said, "You're working from the moment you erupt out of bed in the morning!" And now you can't imagine what my mornings are like. An absolute contrast.

I had been in good health and was in a belly-dance troupe. I dropped out of the troupe only because I was too busy writing a seafood cookbook. My husband and I used to go hiking once or twice a year. But even the thought of going on a hike is too much for me now. I'm a lot more sedentary than before. What we do for fun now is rent a video or go to a movie. I used to socialize so much; I used to have big dinner parties and I would cook all day long. I was told by a lot of people that they really looked forward to coming to dinner at our house because it was always so good. Now I do a lot of frozen casseroles—here I am, a cookbook author, and I don't even cook that often.

My main ability to cope, though, comes from my opioid medications. Initially, I was on the narcotic Percocet. I found myself becoming tolerant. For about three years, I was never prescribed enough. I lived from pill to pill, not in anticipation of getting "high," but in anticipation of the next hour's worth of pain relief. Then I'd have to wait three hours until I could take the next one. My doctor was hesitant to prescribe adequate pain relief because at the time the Washington State Medical Board allowed doctors to prescribe narcotics for nonmalignant pain, but at the same time they were told if they did they could lose their license to practice medicine.

Finally, I changed primary care physicians. My new doctor offered to help me try to control my pain and wasn't afraid to prescribe opioids. I started out on a combination of Oxycodone and acetaminophen, but I was really concerned about liver toxicity. So we went to straight Oxycodone. For a while, it worked. I believe I was already too tolerant to Oxycodone because I had taken it for several years. It didn't really work in the long run; that's why we tried other medications, to find something that was really right for me.

I tried using Duragesic, a narcotic pain patch. I started at the low dose, which is what doctors do, and then they gradually increase the dosage to find your proper amount. The patch is supposed to work for three days. I had to put a plastic film over the three-by-five-inch patch, because it comes off if you get it wet in the shower. But even with the plastic, I couldn't take a bath. And it was hard to find a flat place on my body to put it so it wouldn't come off. I had just my lower hip area and my chest. I'm very narrow there, so I had to alternate the patch site. The patch was so irritating to my skin that it caused eruptions. Then I wouldn't have a place without eruptions to put the next patch on, because it took a while for my skin to heal.

This sounds funny now, but it wasn't funny at the time. I could not get the adhesive from the patch off my skin. It was like a dirty little window frame. The pharmacist suggested peanut butter. I tried mineral oil. I tried mayonnaise. Nobody knew how to get that adhesive off, and I thought, "This is just crazy." I scratched my skin with my fingernail and made even more sores. I met a woman who was on the patch, too, and she said her physical therapist used a cotton square that was an adhesive remover. I went to a local medical supply company and found I could buy a box of individual packets of adhesive remover.

But then the patch didn't release the medication for three days. I called the manufacturer. They said the absorption rate depends on the type of skin you have. Ideally, it's supposed to work for three days, but in reality it only works for one or two days. So I got my doctor to allow me to change the patch more often, which created an even bigger problem with the sores. I wasn't satisfied with the way the patches kept coming off, and I couldn't wear certain clothing; otherwise, the patch would show.

When I had just about had it, my doctor called me and said the pharmacy had contacted her and asked her to try something less expensive (the patches are very expensive, and for the rest of your life, that's a lot of money). We tried methadone instead, and that's what works for me. I'm so pleased.

Initially, I was too drowsy and I didn't like it. But I'd rather be too drowsy than writhing in agony twenty-four hours a day. Methadone lasts longer in the bloodstream than other narcotics. I take methadone around the clock. I also use morphine for breakthrough pain.

On a scale of one to ten, my pain was a twelve before. Now I would say it fluctuates between seven and eight. I'm in pain right now; the methadone doesn't completely take it away. And my doctor and I both agreed that we wouldn't ever be able to completely take it away, but life would be much more tolerable with medication. I am less drowsy and not as nauseous as I used to be. I always have something going on that distracts me from the other pain. Today it's a muscle in my chest and my cheekbone. But it can be my arm or my leg tomorrow—it's always something.

I never made much money before I was hurt. I always called my husband my benefactor. But I was just getting to the point in my writing career where I was starting to make money. I don't know where I would be today if I hadn't been injured. All that stopped. As far as how my husband and I cope financially, it's been more difficult because commercial fishing [which my husband does] is a dying industry. So it's been hard, and equally difficult is the knowledge that I can't help out as much as I want to.

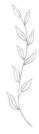

Being ill has turned me into a different person in many ways. I used to be a morning person, and I still haven't gotten over the absolute guilt of lying in bed until late. In my family, you got up, you worked hard, and you went to bed early. And now I'm kind of the opposite. I'm an evening person, because I have to do things when I feel like it. My husband gets upset with me when it's time for him to go to bed and the author in me is just starting to write. But I have to do it when I can.

I'm coping better now, but it's taken me ten years to finally realize I don't have to hide my pain anymore. Still, it is difficult. People want you to be healthy. They don't want you to say that you're ill, unless they think they're God's gift to the ill person and they know how to cure you, even though they don't even know what FM is. It's really annoying.

On a more spiritual level, I think I've become more intuitive, more caring about other people who have pain in their lives, because I can certainly relate better now. I felt like I needed to have some hope and not just focus on the dark times, so I asked myself, "How have I changed, what have I learned?" I was so pleased to know that I had learned something from this experience. This pain, while no blessing, may yet be God's road to enlightenment.

■ Medical Marijuana

Green Cross

Since 1992, Joanna McKee and Stich Miller, cofounders of Green Cross, have provided medical marijuana to patients with a doctor's recommendation in the state of Washington. Voters in that state overwhelmingly passed a medical-marijuana reform initiative in 1998.

They say they're on a mission from God. For the last seven years, Joanna McKee and Stich Miller have risked their property, their health, and their freedom so that they could distribute medical marijuana to sick people. Joanna, who uses medical marijuana to help her deal with chronic pain and muscle spasms that she suffers due to a serious automobile accident, saw a television documentary on the use of medical marijuana to combat the "wasting syndrome" associated with late-stage AIDS. Despite the threat of arrest, prosecution, and jail time, she made the decision to grow and distribute marijuana for herself and others with chronic illnesses.

Just in the last few years, new information has appeared that shows that marijuana can be useful to treat a wide variety of physical problems. Clinical trials are currently being conducted in San Francisco to study the plant's efficacy. The newly published book *Cannabis Indications: Scientific Aspects of Medical Marihuana*, by Martin Martinez [see Bibliography], provides a long list of conditions whose symptoms have been scientifically proven to improve with the controlled use of marijuana, including the following:

- addiction

- AIDS (to treat wasting syndrome and for pain relief)

- anorexia

- arthritis

- asthma

- chemotherapy side effects

- constipation

- diabetes

- digestive disorders

- epilepsy

- glaucoma

- hypertension

- insomnia

- intestinal cramps

191

- menstrual cramps

- migraines

- multiple sclerosis

- muscle spasms

- neuralgia

- premenstrual syndrome

- spasticity

- stroke

In addition to providing medical marijuana (given free of charge if the patient doesn't have the financial means to give a donation), Green Cross will also give the patient four marijuana plant cuttings to grow for their own personal use. Stich dispenses growing tips and supplies as needed. A spin-off service, Compassion in Action, delivers the medical marijuana to the disabled and other people who have difficulty making the trip to pick up their supply of medicine.

Their patients are walking testimonials to the medical benefits of marijuana. One of the co-op's regular customers, Mark K., testifies to the plant's healing powers. "It's been like a wonder drug for me," Mark says. "I've used it for twenty years, ever since I broke my back. Being in a wheelchair is very hard on your body. But I don't hurt in my hips anymore like I used to. I don't need sleep medication anymore. I do take methadone for the pain, but when I use marijuana I don't need nearly as much methadone. It helps me function with my kids a lot better." Members of the local school board weren't as sympathetic, however, and called the Department of Social and Health Services when they found out. "The state took my daughter away because I was using pot for pain," Mark says. "I had to petition the court to get my own daughter back."

In May 1995, Joanna and Stich were arrested by a federal drug task force. One hundred sixty-four marijuana plants were confiscated. The raid surprised even the local police department, which had been practicing a "don't ask, don't tell" policy for more than a year. No one was more surprised than Bainbridge Island Police Chief John Sutton, who learned of the federal action against Green Cross an hour before the search warrant was served. "Marijuana is against the law, and that's our policy," Sutton says. "But I made the decision that we were not going to actively pursue these people. I don't want to say that we turned the other cheek. We simply didn't pursue the matter." Joanna spent the night in jail and was released on her own recognizance; it took Stich two days to get bail. The case was eventually thrown out on the grounds that the evidence was confiscated under an illegal search warrant.

"To a person with chemotherapy-induced nausea, marijuana is a miracle medicine," Tacoma attorney Ralph Seeley told the *Los Angeles Times* after the bust. "[This type of nausea] is not just an upset tummy; it is a violent attack on your system." Seeley campaigned vigorously for marijuana reform initiatives in Washington State but died just months before passage of I-692, which legalized the use of medical marijuana for people with a doctor's recommendation.

Clayton Wilbanks, a Green Cross patient with AIDS and hepatitis, said he feared arrest himself after the federal raid on the co-op. However, he said he would not hesitate to come to Joanna's and Stich's defense: "I was not raised to sit in the back of the bus. I may lose my house, I may lose my freedom, but I'm going to go on the witness stand and testify about the medical benefits of marijuana."

After ten years of an international "War on Drugs" effort, the federal government appears to be finally softening its stance toward marijuana, at least for medicinal purposes. In a stunning reversal of policy, the Clinton administration has allowed government-grown marijuana to be sold to privately funded scientists. The policy change means that clinical trials can begin without having to be funded out of scarce grant money from the National Institutes of Health.

The decision was issued as a regulation by the National Institute on Drug Abuse and is supported by the nation's "drug czar," Barry McCaffrey. The decision comes two months after a study by the Insti-

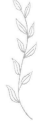

tute of Medicine (a branch of the National Academy of Sciences) con-
cluded that the active ingredients in marijuana appear to be useful for
treating pain, nausea, and severe weight loss associated with AIDS. A
similar review two years earlier reached the same conclusion.

A recent study conducted by researchers at the University of California, Irvine, indicated that medical marijuana has been helpful in
treating schizophrenia in clinical trials. Their findings, published in
the journal *Neuroreport*, reported that high levels of a cannabis-like
chemical were found in the cerebrospinal fluid of schizophrenic
patients. Researchers believe the body may produce the chemical,
anandamine, to fight the disease. The marijuana-like chemical helps
reduce production of dopamine, which has long been suspected to be
a cause of schizophrenia.

Despite state voters' initiatives that allow growing and possessing
marijuana for medical purposes (80 percent of San Francisco voters
voted to legalize medicinal use of marijuana), recent years have seen
more federal action against buyer's co-ops in San Francisco and Oakland, California. Bruce Stubbs, Seattle spokesperson for the federal
Drug Enforcement Agency, reminded the *Los Angeles Times* that federal law prohibits possession of marijuana, even for medical purposes.
"We seriously question whether these 'clubs' are clubs," he said. "They
mostly look like dope traffickers to us."

Public outrage has since forced the DEA to back off from these
organizations. In the last few years, American voters have overwhelmingly passed initiatives allowing for medical marijuana use in seven
states: Alaska, Arizona, California, Colorado, Nevada, Oregon, and
Washington. It is believed that a similar initiative passed in the District of Columbia in 1998; however, the results of the vote have
never been released to the public. Even former Speaker of the House
Newt Gingrich, a conservative Republican, sponsored H.R. 4498, the
Marijuana Therapeutic Act. "It seemed like the right thing to do," he
told reporters.

An early medical-marijuana initiative, I-685, failed in Washington
state in 1997—many say because it also contained provisions to release
marijuana offenders from jail. A scaled-back version gathered enough

signatures and was passed by 60 percent of Washington voters in November 1998. Since then, Green Cross has experienced a tremendous growth in its patient base. "We have three or four doctors calling a day," Stich says. "We've taken on a hundred new patients just in the last few months." They currently serve about 500 patients.

Medical marijuana is obviously not without its detractors. It is still very controversial, and even in states with medical-marijuana laws, its use is heavily regulated. "In Oregon, you have to register your crop with the police department," Stich says. "Like you're a sex offender." Another Green Cross patient, Patty Z., says that the Port Angeles sheriff's office sent deputies to her house in January 1999 to confiscate her medical marijuana. Despite her doctor's recommendation, despite the clearly labeled Green Cross containers, her medicine was taken away by deputy sheriffs who wrote her a receipt for the marijuana and told her she would never see it again. "They didn't arrest me; they didn't charge me with anything," Patty says. "They just walked in, said they didn't need a search warrant, took my medicine, and left."

Battling the DEA and negative public opinion isn't the worst of Green Cross's problems. Someone recently stole almost five thousand dollars' worth of medical marijuana from Green Cross. The burglars didn't take the TV, the VCR, the stereo, the microwave, or the mini-refrigerator. "They knew what they were after," Stich says. He believes it was either an employee or a patient of Green Cross who stole the medicine, as they knew exactly where it was kept. Security has since been beefed up to prevent someone from stealing the needed medicine again.

Joanna, who wears an eyepatch embroidered with a marijuana leaf, believes that this is a holy war and will eventually be won. Although she was initially afraid that the 1998 Washington initiative would fail, she remained strong in the knowledge that they were doing the right thing. "With two civil-rights lawyers in heaven, how could we lose?" she asks, referring to Ralph Seeley and Judith Seeley, two medical-marijuana activists who maintained the courage of their convictions, yet died of cancer while awaiting legalization. Stich and Joanna say they will never give up their fight. In February 1999, they received the

195

"Freedom Fighter of the Month" award from *High Times* magazine. Thanks to dedicated people like the Seeleys, Stich says, "Marijuana is no longer a dirty word."

A Patient's Story: Annie D.

Annie D. is a thirty-seven-year-old who lives in Seattle, Washington. She worked in the computer industry before she was injured in a car accident. Her boyfriend of five years takes care of her financial obligations while she awaits disability benefits. Narcotic painkillers and medical marijuana have helped her to fight the symptoms of her FM and CFS.

In January 1996, I was driving to work on a cold, gray, drizzly day. Two cars in front of me suddenly braked. I, too, slowed down, and had just rolled to a complete stop when behind me came the sound of *screech-wham!* I had been rear-ended. The woman who hit me told me that she already had one at-fault accident and wanted to take care of this without involving her insurance company. There seemed to be minimal damage to the car (you can't kill a Volkswagen), and I didn't feel like I was hurt, so I agreed to not call the police. Bad decision. Yet how could I have known then that this one incident would so radically and irrevocably change my life?

For as long as I can remember, I've prepared for literary success. In 1986, when I was twenty-three, I went to college (after working two jobs to save up enough money). I worked part-time and work-study jobs for four years in order to support myself while getting a bachelor's degree in journalism. For the last year and a half of my college career, I served as columnist and copy editor for the college newspaper—receiving scholarships and a summer internship. I graduated in 1989 with straight As in my core courses and moved to Asheville, North Carolina, where I received international attention and accolades for my reporting.

I relocated to Seattle in 1992, where I wrote for a local independent newspaper from 1992 to 1994. My publisher, fellow reporter, and

I were awarded the national 1994 Investigative Reporters & Editors award for best investigative series—a coveted award usually given to *Time, Newsweek,* and other prestigious national news publications. In May 1995, I took a technical writing job with a software company. My ultimate career goal was to be able to head my own publishing company by the age of forty-five.

Now, because of the accident injuries and subsequent FM and CFS, those dreams are no longer available to me. It feels like all my hard work has been for nothing. The mere act of typing this has the muscles in my arms, shoulders, and neck spasming painfully. I am no longer able to put in twelve-hour days at the computer, a requisite in today's publishing environment. Before the accident, I was able to earn a comfortable living and do pretty much whatever I wanted, whenever I wanted to. Life was good. Then I was hit and, in an instant, poof, all my life plans were gone.

A little more than a year after the accident, and only two months after I was diagnosed with FM and had to permanently reduce my workload, I was fired from my job. I was thirty-five years old and had never been fired from a job in my life. I was devastated and was very sick for two months after the firing. I developed a terrible cold, which turned into bronchitis, which turned into bronchospasms that required steroidal inhalants to cure. My entire system just shut down. I spent my thirty-sixth birthday at the welfare office, trying to apply for benefits. My FM physician filled out the paperwork for me and indicated that I might never be able to work full-time again. After the office visit, I sat in his parking lot and cried.

I suffered needlessly for two years because my doctor refused to prescribe anything more than anti-inflammatories. The narcotic I take now, Oxycontin, has allowed me some relief from the unending pain I've lived with since the accident. Being on narcotics isn't all joy and happiness, though. I frequently have nausea and vomiting, especially if I have been in a noisy environment. If I forget to take it for even a couple of hours, I become very anxious and sick to my stomach. Constipation is a constant companion, too, and I worry that I will have to be on narcotics for the rest of my life. Still, if I weren't taking nar-

197

cotic painkillers, I couldn't function at all. I also use medical marijuana for my pain and muscle spasms.

I am no longer able to participate in virtually any of the activities that once brought me so much pleasure. Every aspect of my life has been affected. I am not able to be as sexually intimate with my boyfriend as I once was. Our relationship has suffered, since much of the financial burden of keeping our home (in which we have lived for more than four years) has fallen on him. Now, after working all day, he comes home and has to take care of most of the housework because I am unable to do it. I used to enjoy cooking and experimenting with different types of cuisine (Vietnamese and curries were among our favorites). Now dinner frequently comes from a can.

Good days are few and far between. On bad days, I hurt so much I can't think of anything else. It hurts to stand, to walk, to sit. Some nights, it even hurts to lay my head on my pillow. It's hard to plan anything, as I never know from one morning to the next how I will feel that day. One morning, my neck and shoulder muscles will drive me crazy. Then, after a few days, that pain will inexplicably disappear, only to reappear as severe leg cramps after I return from a walk. The next day, I'll have severe stomach cramps and diarrhea. At times, the pain and misery have been so bad that I didn't want to go on living.

I've learned so much through all of this. You have to be your own advocate, you have to be persistent, and you have to be aggressive in order to get the care you need. Ironic, isn't it, that we are forced to be strong at a time when we feel more tired and weak than we ever have before. HMOs and insurance companies try every trick in the book to delay you, as they count on you either dying or giving up before they will be forced to pay up. It's your health and well being that are at stake; if you aren't willing to stand up for your rights, who will?

Remember the old joke by Henny Youngman? "Guy goes to the doctor, raises his arm, and says, 'Doc, it hurts when I do this.' Doctor says, 'Don't do that!'" We know it isn't that easy, but we can all learn a lighthearted lesson from that silly joke. Discontinue what causes pain (excessive exercising, strenuous yoga, working full-time, carrying heavy grocery bags, etc.). Our stomachs are upset, our legs and arms hurt, our heads are pounding, but we can be strong in the face of adversity. We can find other ways of living. We have to, if we are to survive. It is our responsibility to demand the care that we deserve. I am lucky to have finally found a pain-management specialist willing to prescribe narcotics to help me handle the pain. I am a firm believer in better living through chemicals.

Chapter 12

The Future of Fibromyalgia and Chronic Fatigue Syndrome

O UR GOAL THROUGHOUT THIS BOOK has been to explore new treatment options. More research is being done and more information becomes available on FM and CFS every day. Researchers continue to explore the role of Substance P, the relationship between chlamydia pneumoniae and CFS, sleep disorders in FM and CFS, and viral infections and CFS, just to name a few areas of interest. The studies discussed in this chapter are only a handful of the dozens going on all across the country. As research progresses, new theories attempt to explain how these symptoms develop, and researchers are trying to use that new knowledge to find a cure.

The latest research on FM indicates that it is predominantly a neurotransmitter disorder. Since neurotransmitters are regulated by the body during sleep, researchers are studying sleep disturbances.

Mari participated in one such study at a local university in 1997.

She slept at the lab for three continuous nights; she had her blood drawn throughout the night and wore a device that monitored her activity during sleep. She also had to stop taking her medications for several weeks so that they would not interfere with the study's findings. Despite the inconveniences, Mari says she wanted to be part of the study because she felt it was an invaluable tool that might eventually help others. "It was surprisingly easy to sleep in the lab," she says—even with all the electrodes attached with sticky stuff all over her face and in her hair.

One of the people interviewed for this chapter, University of Washington researcher Dr. Carol Landis, has begun to investigate prolactin and its role in stimulating the immune system. Reports by a group of researchers in Europe indicate that if you give certain peptides or stimulants to patients, the brain can be triggered to secrete increased amounts of prolactin at different times of the day. "When they've done that to subjects with FM," Dr. Landis says, "there was a slight increase in the secretion of prolactin from the pituitary. We were actually expecting we might see an increase in prolactin at night compared to our age-matched controls, but we found quite the contrary."

Other research currently being conducted focuses on how people with chronic pain cope, and examines ways treatment can better serve such people. One researcher we interviewed, Dr. Dennis Turk, says that people with chronic pain cope in different ways: "We have looked at people who have back pain, chronic headaches, temporomandibular joint disorders or facial pain, metastatic cancer, and regional cancer." In each of those different medical populations, Dr. Turk has identified three subgroups of patients:

1. "dysfunctional" patients

2. "interpersonally distressed" individuals

3. "adaptive copers"

The research data implies that, independent of the medical diagnosis, there are different ways that individuals adapt to pain, Dr. Turk explains. "Individuals who have FM differ in their response, depend-

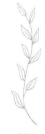

ing upon their psychosocial patterns."

According to the March/April 1999 issue of *The CFIDS Chronicle*, the co-enzyme NADH has been shown to reduce fatigue symptoms in clinical trials. NADH is the reduced form of nicotinamide adenine dinucleotide, which is a naturally occurring co-enzyme that triggers energy production in cells by generating ATP (adenosine triphosphate). ATP stores energy in the body's cells. If cellular levels of NADH are depleted, brain and muscle cells lose their ability to function effectively. As NADH levels rise in the body, researchers believe, the cells become more energized which makes the body feel stronger.

In a double-blind placebo-controlled crossover study of 26 patients with CFS, Dr. Joseph Bellanti and colleagues reported that eight patients improved during the four weeks they were taking NADH, while only two patients improved while on placebo. In a continuation of the study in which all volunteers were knowingly taking the NADH supplement called Enada, 72 percent reported significant improvement in fatigue with no severe adverse affects. Initial results of the study have been published in the February 1999 issue of the *Annals of Allergy, Asthma and Immunology*.

The new trend in treatment of FM and CFS is self-management. This simply means that patients take an active role in their own healing by educating themselves and using a variety of behavioral techniques. (In her interview for this chapter, Dr. Kate Lorig outlines specific self-management techniques that the patient can use as a means of supplementing their doctors' care.) Self-management is a way to empower oneself when there appear to be few available treatment options. This technique emphasizes the partnership between patient and provider.

Although researchers are searching for a cure, many of the people we interviewed for this book who are surviving on a day-to-day basis say they wonder whether the day of a miracle cure will ever come. While some say they feel a sense of optimism about their future, others don't have that faith. Andrea says she probably wouldn't be able to get out of bed in the morning if she didn't hold onto the hope that someday researchers will find that cure. Mari doesn't even allow herself to dream of a cure, because the pain seems to be such a big part of her that it's impossible to visualize life without it. "Having the pain just miraculously go away seems so far-fetched to me," she says. "For me, healing is every day, not in the future."

Until these studies give us the answers and the cure we're demanding, the best we can do is try to alleviate some of the symptoms of FM and CFS. We must remain confident that one day there will be a cure and we will again be able to return to the lives we knew before, free of pain and exhaustion.

Self-Management Techniques

Kate Lorig, Ph.D.

Dr. Kate Lorig holds a doctorate in public health and is the director of the Patient Education Research Center at the Stanford University School of Medicine.

My center tries to help people with all kinds of musculoskeletal problems, not just FM or CFS. We teach people with chronic illnesses, whether it's FM or diabetes or any other illness. Anyone with a chronic illness needs to learn that there is often a three-part approach to healing. There's the medical treatment. There's surgical treatment (which is not terribly relevant for people with FM and CFS). The third is the behavioral aspect. Anyone with a chronic illness needs to be making day-to-day decisions and doing day-to-day problem solving. Like any other chronic illness, FM and CFS are things that will never be cured, and how well one lives with the condition depends a great deal on day-to-day self-management.

I try to help people learn self-management techniques. It's like having a toolbox; you teach people to use all kinds of tools. We don't expect them to use every tool every day. They may never need to use some of these tools. It's like the wrench I've had in my house for twenty years and never used until one day I had a leaky faucet. Self-management

203

means having the tools and knowing when to use them appropriately.

One of the things we know about people who are good self-managers, who have confidence, skills, and necessary knowledge, is that they are more physically and socially active, they have fewer symptoms, and they live more productive lives. It's not simply a matter of behavior modification or medication. The best treatment is a combination of both.

One of those skills is exercise. I don't think it makes much difference what exercise people do. *Chi kung* is fine. *Tai chi* is fine. Walking is fine. Some people love Feldenkrais (a movement therapy), and some people don't. But the idea that one needs to keep one's body physically fit is one of the key behavioral self-management techniques. This is more a matter of pacing than of mere exercise. Follow some simple rules: If you have more pain when you finish than when you started, you probably did too much, and you need to do a bit less next time. Exercise can be broken into little tiny bits. You can do five minutes three times a day, or ten minutes twice a day; you don't have to do one big bout. Exercise and staying in good general condition are two of the main things we stress.

There's a whole set of pain-management techniques, such as self-talk or visual imagery, that help patients deal with problems such as pain and fatigue. Again, there is no one thing that is better than another. Simple things such as distraction techniques, like counting backward from one hundred by threes, can work as well as those that take time and consistent practice, like some meditation techniques do. It all depends on how much people are willing to do, how much effort they are willing to put into it. Any chronic illness, not just FM or CFS, has a whole psychological overlay that includes anger, fear, frustration, or depression. Those things are normal; they happen because people suddenly face an altered existence. These are things that go along with any chronic illness. Some good studies have been done that show the emotional overlay of chronic illness. All the things that one had hoped and planned for may not be possible anymore. You need to learn how to cope with that.

Many self-management techniques, like exercise, help you deal with these emotions. Sometimes medications are also necessary. Unfortunately, people with FM and CFS tend to get labeled with a mental-illness stigma. I'm not exactly sure why that is; probably because it's so difficult to document any organic damage.

Antidepressants are useful and can be prescribed for two reasons. One of the major problems for people with FM or CFS is inability to get enough rest and decent sleep. Antidepressants are very good for that. We also use them for all kinds of pain syndromes, not just for FM. People end up personalizing, though, sometimes beyond what is rational, and may be hesitant to take drugs they perceive as being only used for people with mental-health issues. People with FM and CFS need to start thinking of themselves as having a chronic illness, and they need to deal with FM or CFS like any other chronic illness.

The future is very unpredictable for people with chronic illness, because they don't know how they're going to feel day to day. I also hear people say, "No one understands me, nobody can help me, I feel terrible, and I'm going to sit home and feel sorry for myself." They've just given up. Anybody with a chronic illness has to learn how to manage their illness in order to be able to have any quality of life for themselves.

Psychological Aspects of Chronic Pain

Dr. Dennis Turk

Dr. Dennis Turk is the John and Emma Bonica Professor of Anesthesiology and Pain Research at the University of Washington. He is also director of the university's FM Research Center. He is an adjunct professor of psychiatry at the University of Pittsburgh in Pennsylvania.

Fibromyalgia is a broad term that, in my opinion, probably describes people with different physical and psychological characteristics. Very likely, there are subgroups of people who have different sets of characteristics. A problem with treating FM patients as a homogeneous set of individuals is that we have probably provided some people with

205

treatments that are appropriate and some that are not. If we want to understand FM and provide better treatment, we really need to subdivide or classify subgroups of individuals with this particular diagnosis.

A lot of FM research uses a heterogeneous group of patients but treats them as if they were a homogenous group. In doing so, we may be offering inappropriate treatment to patients. When we look into the literature on treatment options, the confusion we see over and over again is that some treatments seem to be beneficial to some patients but not to others. Very likely, when we give the same treatment to all individuals, we are providing appropriate treatment for only a small subset of patients. When you try to replicate these findings, what originally looked like promising results don't appear to recur, because we are missing the treatment boat. I use the analogy of advising a patient to take multivitamins when there is simply a vitamin B deficiency. You would be better off prescribing only vitamin B to that individual rather than giving them a whole range of multivitamins and hoping they are going to get the vitamin B they need.

To truly treat a chronic pain state like FM, we need to consider several areas of assessment. The biomedical or medical domain includes factors associated with physiology, anatomy, and biochemistry. The second axis or domain is the psychosocial domain; that is, how does the presence of these symptoms impact people's lives? And the third domain or axis is the behavioral axis, which is how people respond to the presence of this set of symptoms. We need to base treatment on this multiaxial assessment of pain, including these three areas. To date, the research I have been involved with tries to identify subgroups of patients based on how they are coping and adapting to the presence of their symptoms. That taps into the second and third domains, the psychosocial and behavioral aspects. This in no way suggests that I believe psychological factors cause the symptoms, but rather suggests that when individuals have lived with these symptoms for long periods of time, they develop different responses to their problems.

To appropriately treat people, we must pay attention to physical signs as well as psychosocial and behavioral signs. In future research, we hope to subdivide patients based on the physical factors that may contribute to their symptoms. I am optimistic that we will ultimately have what I call "dual diagnosis." We will then have a medical diagnosis that includes psychosocial factors (the way pain affects people's lives, how they adjust to that, and how it affects their behavior).

We currently are conducting studies demonstrating that there are, in fact, at least three different subgroups of patients with FM, based on psychosocial and behavioral factors and how individuals adapt to their situation and their set of symptoms. The three subgroups we identified were based on statistical means of analyzing people's responses to a questionnaire. We asked questions about the impact of pain on individuals' lives, how they respond to it, how much control they feel they have over their lives, and how much impact their illnesses have had on their actual activities.

These three subgroups consist of the following:

- The first subgroup we refer to as "dysfunctional." These individuals have high levels of pain and emotional distress. They feel they have little control over their lives and tend to be inactive.

- The second group we refer to as "interpersonally distressed." These individuals also have high levels of pain, and have somewhat higher levels of emotional distress than other patients. What is unique about them is their perception of how significant others or people in their environment respond to them. Despite the fact that they have pain symptoms like those of the dysfunctional group, they feel they get very little support from significant people and a lot of negative responses.

- The third group we call "adaptive copers." These people, despite the symptoms of FM, appear to be functioning and coping relatively well. Their lives are as impacted as those of other patients, but they tend to remain active.

We currently have funding from the National Institute of Arthritis, Musculoskeletal Diseases and Skin Diseases to see if we can directly evaluate the matching of different types of treatments based on those patient characteristics, so that every patient will receive some level of physical therapy. We will also try to match the treatment to the psychosocial behavioral characteristics. By doing this type of intervention, we hope to be able to identify which patients with what characteristics are most likely to benefit from particular types of interventions. We anticipate that we will then be able to start matching patients with particular characteristics, both physical and psychological, to specific treatments.

We are just beginning this five-year project, so we aren't yet able to say whether we will achieve the treatment responses we hope to. We have shown that there are definitely different patient responses to treatments, based on their psychosocial characteristics. Over time, we will be able to develop better interventions that will be more closely matched to the patient's individual characteristics.

We are trying to understand these individuals and find the best type of treatment for them. The hope is that eventually we will be able to assess groups of FM patients and give each of them a dual diagnosis, which will be a combination of a biomedical diagnosis and a psychosocial behavioral diagnosis.

In five years, we hope to identify the best treatment for these individuals on the psychosocial side, but also on the medical/biomedical side. Let me reiterate that, although I have used the term "psychosocial" and "behavioral," there is no suggestion that psychological factors cause FM or CFS symptoms. Rather, when someone has to cope with these types of symptoms over long periods of time, they begin having an impact, psychologically, socially, and physically. As individuals, we all experience life in all different dimensions, and so we really want to treat people as a whole person, not just an arm or a leg or a tender point.

▧ Sleep Dysfunction and Fibromyalgia

Carol A. Landis, D.N.Sc.

Carol A. Landis is a professor at the University of Washington research-ing sleep dysfunction. Her study on sleep dysfunction, funded by the National Institute of Nursing Research, looks at sleep and nighttime hormone patterns in middle-aged women with FM. The purpose of her research is to find new ways to help regulate hormonal imbalances that may cause or contribute to excessive pain in people with FM.

Waking up and feeling unrefreshed is a complaint that's long been part of the symptomatology of FM, but we don't yet understand very well what is disordered about their sleep. Some women with FM may have a particular sleep disorder—sleep apnea, for example—and treating the sleep apnea can certainly help with daytime sleepiness and fatigue.

I am currently exploring sleep and hormones in women and how they may impact FM. There are two hormones, growth hormone and prolactin, that are clearly sleep related. For example, it's long been known that when you stay up all night and are sleep deprived, the amounts of growth hormone and prolactin in your body go down. With FM, women don't sleep as well as their age-matched controls. Their sleep efficiencies were measured at close to 85 percent, but they had a nighttime excretion of growth hormone and prolactin similar to what a normal person would have if you kept him or her up all night. It looks like a sleep-deprivation pattern. And we don't really have an explanation for that at present.

We carefully screen our control subjects so that they are good sleep-ers without symptoms, and then we compare them to women with FM. All the patients who come into the clinic are screened for eligi-bility. Each of the patients in the clinic who meets our eligibility cri-teria is then contacted by the research nurse. If they meet our other eligibility requirements, they begin keeping a month-long journal of daily symptoms. We do that because we are interested in tracking how the symptoms fluctuate over time rather than relying totally on the

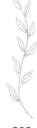

209

patient's memory. The journal asks the patient to answer a series of questions on a scale from zero to four for various types of symptoms they have throughout the day. And it's not geared just toward the musculoskeletal system, but all the different body systems. We also ask people to record the time they go to bed, the time they get up, how many hours they slept, how well they slept, how stressful their day is, and the types of medications they take.

When the diaries are completed, they are mailed here to the sleep lab, and our research nurse scans the diaries to see if they meet further eligibility criteria. We then set up an initial telephone screening interview for individuals who are experiencing pain and discomfort greater than four on a scale of zero to ten. We track their symptoms for a month, then we look at that diary data to determine if they have pain for more than a week in a month. And if they are eligible at that point, we set up an individual protocol for weaning them off medications that could alter their sleep. The medications we are most interested in excluding are analgesics, antidepressants, and sedatives. To participate in the study, our subjects must to be willing to come off their medications. Getting people to give up their medications has been very difficult. But the only way we can get a handle on what's happening during sleep is if women don't take medications that alter their nighttime sleep patterns, and likely alter their nighttime hormone patterns as well.

In the sleep lab, we draw blood to ensure that people have an adequate amount of red blood cells, because we do all-night blood draws on the third night of the study. We monitor their activity; we monitor their sleep; we screen them for whether they have a particular sleep disorder like sleep apnea or restless leg syndrome. On the first night, we study them while they are adapting to the lab environment. On the second night, we study them for what we call our "baseline sleep night," and then the third night of the study, we draw blood each hour from 8 P.M. until 7 A.M.

On the second day of the study, we have them collect their urine for twenty-four hours, because we're interested in looking at certain hormones that are excreted over that period of time. We also do a blood draw on the morning after they've slept in the lab for the second night, because we're looking at some parameters of immune function. We also measure their serotonin levels. Other researchers have proven that the sleep of people with FM is disordered; however, we're expanding to other areas that researchers haven't explored prior to this study.

We've begun some preliminary analysis, and I presented data at the Society for Neuroscience last fall which shows that at night women experience reduced levels of growth hormones and prolactin. The decreased growth hormone was somewhat predictable, based on work that Robert Bennett, M.D., has done at Oregon Health Sciences University. Some years ago, they reported that a peripheral hormone made by the liver called "insulin-like growth factor"—and the production of that hormone in the periphery—is in part regulated by the production of growth hormone from the pituitary. The major surge of growth hormone during a twenty-four-hour period occurs during the first three to five hours of sleep at night. Our subjects with FM have considerably reduced amounts of growth hormone compared to our age-matched controls. And we've also found, quite unexpectedly, that the women have reduced levels of prolactin as well. Prolactin is a hormone that is very important in lactation. At the end of pregnancy, there is a surge of prolactin secretion in preparation for lactation. In general, women tend to secrete more prolactin than men.

We researchers have found FM to be an intriguing and interesting disorder. Again, it's most certainly a woman's disorder. Reduced prolactin might help explain why more women than men have FM. But there's so much more to learn about the disorder than we know now. At present, women are being treated for their symptoms, but it's obvious that these treatments are not very effective, because women are still having trouble managing their symptoms. I don't think we know enough about FM to be able to predict what therapies would work best for all FM sufferers. It may well be that there are certain subtypes or subgroups of individuals with FM, some of whom might respond to one type of therapy better than another. Without further research, it's hard to predict at this time what those treatments might be.

211

New Directions in Chronic Fatigue Syndrome Research

Rich Carson

Once upon a time, Rich Carson was a successful investment specialist. Ten years ago, he became totally disabled with CFS. He subsequently founded the company Pro Health, Inc., which sells herbal and vitamin supplements through the *CFIDS & FM Health Resource Catalog* and via the Internet. He has been referred to as the "leading fundraiser in the country for CFS," having raised more than two million dollars to date.

I am totally disabled with CFS, although I don't have FM, which frequently occurs concurrently with CFS. I had an acute onset of the disease in August 1981 and became totally disabled in July 1987. I was given psychometric tests and an MRI brain scan. The psychometric tests indicated I had had a thirty-point drop in my IQ, and the brain scan showed numerous brain lesions. I was also given a SPECT scan to determine if I had a brain tumor, stroke, or other serious brain abnormality. The results were positive. They found fifty-one small areas on my brain that resembled small strokes, where the tissue appeared to be dead. They also found reduced blood flow to my brain. An EEG test determined I had also developed a brain electrical activity disorder (a sort of epileptic type of disorder made worse by exposure to synthetic substances such as paints or perfumes).

I had heard about a product used to treat low natural killer cell syndrome, which is the name they gave CFS in Japan. Patients in a Japanese research study were treated with LEM, an extract of the mycelium of the edible shiitake mushroom. There was a significant positive response in the vast majority of patients. By coincidence, I came across a product that contained freeze-dried LEM, which had just been introduced into the American marketplace by a company called Source Naturals. I was able to persuade Source Naturals, as well as the manufacturing company in Japan, to donate twenty thousand dollars' worth of LEM for American CFS research. I then contacted researchers for whom I had already been raising money (Drs. Jay Goldstein, Daniel Peterson, Anthony Komaroff, and Paul Cheney) to submit research proposals to test the efficacy of LEM as a natural treatment for CFS patients.

Dr. Goldstein received the bulk of the product and disbursed it to his patients free of charge. Many of these patients had an excellent response. He began prescribing the product, even though it was virtually impossible to find the product in any health-food store in the United States. Patients were supposed to take eighteen tablets a day, which cost two hundred and eighty dollars a month. I was able to get a special deal, and I made the product available to patients at half the price. I donated these profits to the CFIDS Association of America.

At this point, I was doing it pretty much on my own, with the help of my girlfriend. It was just my little baby. Then I came up with the idea of starting a CFS "buyer's club" to increase the availability of LEM and other difficult-to-find specialty products used by the more innovative and aggressive doctors specializing in treating CFS. I had been interviewed in *Rolling Stone* magazine for a two-part piece titled "Journey Into Hell." A number of people, primarily people in the entertainment industry, read my interview and contacted me to donate money. I also had developed a good relationship with Blake Edwards (who has CFS and has been very public about it) and his wife, Julie Andrews.

We produced the first major celebrity fundraiser for CFS. More than sixty people attended, including Tri-Star Pictures President Michael Medevoy, former Minnesota Governor Rudy Purpich, and multimillionaire industrialist Max Palevsky. Numerous other luminaries in the entertainment industry also attended. The keynote speakers were Dr. Paul Cheney, who is arguably the most famous CFS specialist in the United States because of his frequent interviews and outspoken opinions; Dr. Jim Jones, who is one of the fathers of CFS research; and the highly respected Harvard Medical School professor Dr. Anthony Komaroff. From the fundraiser, we were able to raise about two hundred and eighty thousand dollars for CFS research.

Right now, I'm very interested in a virus getting a lot of attention from several of the top CFS researchers. It's called human herpes virus six (HHV6). This virus now appears to be the most likely candidate as the actual cause of CFS and possibly even FM. Dr. Dharam Ablashi, who discovered HHV6 along with virologist Dr. Robert Gallo, presented research findings at the American Association for CFS Conference in Boston in 1998 which indicated that HHV6 seems to be involved in a majority of CFS cases.

Dr. Konstance Knox and Dr. Don Carrigan from the company Wisconsin Viral Research Group, who are probably the world's leading authorities on HHV6, have also been studying the prevalence of active HHV6 in CFS and FM patients. The Knox/Carrigan team has found that two-thirds of CFS patients have this potentially dangerous virus in their bodies in an activated, replicating form at any given time. These researchers are also finding HHV6 in the cerebrospinal fluids of people with CFS. This is very exciting news.

Fortunately, HHV6 is a wimpy virus that people with normal immune systems can handle readily. If a person's immune system is suppressed due to stress, exposure to toxic chemicals, or possibly even because of a genetic weakness in handling viral infections, the HHV6 virus can come out of latency. It then starts to infect and damage the immune system, brain, and other organs. In medical situations where the patient has to be on immunosuppressant drugs, like chemotherapy or organ transplants, it is well documented that HHV6 can be fatal.

With respect to HHV6, I believe we were the first organization in the world to recognize the possible role it might play in these diseases. We decided not only to try to persuade the top HHV6 researchers in the world to take a look at that possibility; we decided to stick our necks out and start raising and donating funds for several other research projects to test that hypothesis. This began about two and a half years ago, and is still gaining momentum. The CFIDS & FM Health Resource began funding a pilot research program in which eight CFS patients were tested: six or seven of them tested positive for active HHV6. I have to emphasize the word "active," because HHV6 is a pretty common virus and is never seen in healthy individuals in its active state.

That's exactly what researchers found when they tested the five healthy control subjects and numerous nonpatients since then. None of these subjects had any HHV6 activity whatsoever. The researchers at Wisconsin Viral Research Group use a technique they invented to test for the virus called the rapid culture technique. I believe they are currently the only ones in the world that know how to test for active HHV6. The beauty of this technique, from a diagnostic point of view, is that it determines whether the virus is actually replicating at the time your blood is taken. If you can culture a live virus out of someone's blood, then there's no doubt they have the virus.

Dr. Knox says she is finding a very high percentage of FM patients with active HHV6, the most drug-resistant virus of the eight known herpes family of viruses. I am excited because researchers are now testing more than ten different drugs to see if they will kill HHV6 at levels that aren't toxic to patients. These drugs aren't on the market yet but will be soon. I am pretty confident they will find one or a combination of drugs that's going to work. Then *boom!* We're off to the races. This would be the perfect and logical time for the wealthy pharmaceutical industry to start pumping money into CFS and FM research. My goal is to get Corporate America involved, since the government seems to be dragging its heels.

Another thing I'm interested in right now is a new surgical procedure for FM and CFS patients who have chiari malformation. Chiari malformation is not new. What is new is the recognition that FM or CFS patients might actually have it. The National Fibromyalgia Research Association in Salem, Oregon, is funding a study to determine the percentage of FM patients who have chiari malformation or spinal-cord compression. Chiari malformation is a congenital abnormality in the portion of the cerebellum where it is displaced into the spinal canal. This results in spinal-cord or brain-stem compression. The surgical procedure is designed to relieve this compression. It is not a cure, but it is an opportunity for significant improvement. An MRI brain scan is the only way it can be diagnosed, and the scan must be done at exactly the correct angle. This surgical procedure is being performed by several neurosurgeons, including Dr. Daniel Heffez of

Chicago and Dr. Michael Rosner of Charlotte, North Carolina. There is no question that patients are improving, but they continue to have some symptoms.

The CFS Buyer's Club changed its name a few years ago to the CFIDS & FM Health Resource because of the extremely high overlap rate of the two diseases. In fact, some researchers feel that the two are just different forms of the same disease. We still sell all of the supplements and alternative health products beneficial to people with CFS, but we have added several new products for the treatment of FM because of the differences in symptoms. We still donate our profits back to fund medical research, which is the program of which I am most proud. Our recent *Healthwatch* "Best of Ten Years" issue contained an article discussing the HHV6 findings and articles on the latest CFIDS and FM research and treatments. We also included a list of the twenty-five most efficacious supplements for CFIDS and FM patients. *Healthwatch* has helped a lot of people by keeping them informed and giving them hope.

As an individual, I am about getting well and getting as many people well as I possibly can. I want to find an end to the disease that has destroyed so much of my life. It's given me a new identity, one that sometimes I am very happy with. Other times it is very confining, and I feel like I am a prisoner in my own body. My goal is to find the key that will unlock the door, so I can escape from prison and be free to live a normal life again. Frankly, my goal is to put Health Resource out of business. That'll be the happiest day of my life, when my business goes out of business.

Chapter 13

Legal Considerations

KNOWING ABOUT YOUR RIGHTS under Social Security disability law, and knowing what you can expect during the benefits application process, can help you feel a little less apprehensive. This chapter illustrates the need for good legal representation, especially for people who may be disabled by FM or CFS. It is your responsibility to protect your rights under the law. There is still substantial dissent among the medical community and Social Security administrative law judges about FM and CFS. Private insurance companies are adept at exploiting this dissent and the lag time between injury and diagnosis; they will use every method at their disposal to mitigate their financial liability in these situations. Social Security is also suspicious of people who claim they are disabled without having objective data to back up their claims.

Approximately 2 percent of the American population has been diagnosed with FM, according to the American College of Rheumatology; however, it is believed that the actual percentage of sufferers is much higher due to disbelief within the medical community. These naysayers have the power to wreak havoc in an injured person's life. Social Security disability benefits can be difficult if not impossible to receive if a person is not visibly disabled (blind, paralyzed, etc.). There are only a handful of conditions—such as terminal cancer—for which a person is automatically awarded benefits. Everyone else has to go through a lengthy and tedious process of applications, hearings, and appeals. Most attorneys will not accept a case until the person has been denied once. Hiring an attorney at the second level (the reconsideration level) is essential to ensure fair consideration under the law.

Once you have obtained a formal diagnosis of FM or CFS and you believe you are unable to work as a result, you should immediately contact the Social Security Administration [see Resources] to begin the claims process. Be prepared to submit many pages of documentation, including detailed descriptions of your limitations and daily activities. Be prepared to be denied several times before you are successful in your petition for benefits. Of the twenty-seven patients we interviewed for this book who applied for benefits, only two received their benefits the first time they applied. In some cases, this process can take years. Despite the tedious paperwork and rejection, you must persevere if you are to receive the benefits to which you are entitled as a chronically ill person. While you are awaiting your disability determination, you may also be eligible to receive some state or federal welfare benefits. In fact, the Department of Social Services in your community should be able to help you begin your Social Security application process.

Having a reputable physician to back you up is as essential as finding a good attorney to represent you at your disability hearing. Croil Anderson, an attorney specializing in Social Security disability benefits, says, "When you look to the system for benefits, the first question they ask is, 'Are you engaging in any substantial gainful activity?' You can only get benefits if you are unable to engage in any substantial gainful activity for a period of one year or more from a 'medically determinable impairment.' Receiving benefits depends upon what a person has and whether they have a medically determinable impairment. Even though you have the diagnosis of FM, that doesn't automatically mean you win the case. You have to prove that you've been disabled by the illness.

"We recently had some cases where, at the administrative law judge level, it was decided that there was no medically determinable impairment," Croil says. "Then the appeals council—which is the appellate entity above the administrative law judges—said that judge was wrong. Also, there are many federal court cases that have determined that FM is a medically determinable impairment. The problem is that FM is fairly subjective, and some physicians say it is a controversial diagnosis. It is critical to have a qualified physician document your medical treatment over a long period of time. It gets to be very complex in terms of determining who is disabled by this illness and who isn't, but at least in the eyes of Social Security it is becoming an 'acceptable' illness that can disable a person.

"In fact, in April 1999, the Social Security Administration issued Ruling 99-2p, which officially recognizes that CFS and FM are 'medically determinable impairments.' This once and for all answers the question of whether these illnesses can actually contribute to a person not being able to work a normal job. Now, all adjudicators should use the same policies and procedures in determining disability claims for people with CFS and FM. The ruling uses the diagnostic criteria for CFS and FM established by the Centers for Disease Control and American College of Rheumatology. Now, a claimant's case can be determined on an individual basis, which is how it is done in any other medical case.

"When should a person hire an attorney? I think they have to make that call after they've been denied the first time. Whether the attorney takes it at that level will be discussed during the initial consultation. After the first denial, you are asked to fill out a lot of forms, including a daily activities form, a pain form, a chronic fatigue form. They ask you what a typical day in your life is like. All of that has an impact in terms of the ultimate decision made in the case. According to national statistics, approximately 14 percent of people who applied

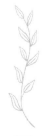

219

won at the reconsideration [second] level. So I never give my client a lot of hope they're going to win at that level; it just isn't there."

We have all had difficulty receiving disability benefits. Private insurance companies are loathe to pay out under long-term disability policies for illnesses that cannot be "proven." There are no X-rays, no blood tests, no urinalyses to back up our claims. The application process through which a person can receive Social Security benefits can take years and wears us down in the meantime. Administrative law judges have a hard time believing that a person who isn't obviously incapacitated, who looks fine, could be unable to hold down even a part-time job on a regular basis.

Many of the people we interviewed for this book live in poverty and were on welfare for years before they were finally successful in their petition for benefits. They've lost their health, their happiness, their ability to earn a living, and their ability to care for themselves; some even lost their homes. "Dealing with my finances has been a real bummer," says Anna K. "I went from seventy thousand dollars a year to zero, and then I was trying to get Social Security for six months. They have to have all these affidavits and all this stuff that everyone who is applying for Social Security has to go through. But that brought in five hundred and eighty-four dollars a month. I was thrilled to have it."

Hilary S. experienced hopelessness first-hand when she tried to get financial help after being hurt in a car accident. "When I initially applied for Social Security disability benefits," she says, "I actually applied before I got the diagnosis. I thought something was seriously wrong with me. But when I first applied, I got denied. I filed for reconsideration and got denied again. I appealed that verdict, went to court, and had a very conservative judge who ripped me apart. My petition was denied a third time. Now I am waiting at the appeal level, which is supposed to take six months. But they're saying it could take up to two years.

"We have requested either to have the decision overturned by a different judge or to get a new hearing by a different judge," Hilary says. "We didn't feel we were going to receive a fair hearing by that judge, and in fact, he did some illegal things in my case. His decision was based upon the fact that he thought it was 'secondary gain' against my car accident settlement. Also, he felt that I would be able to gain a higher level of management in the workforce if I were disabled. He thought it would better my career to be disabled. This makes no sense. Why he thinks that way, I have no clue, because I have not worked for more than three years. And on top of it, he ripped apart some of my health-care providers."

One of the most difficult things Betty M. says she's had to endure was the process of getting disability benefits. "In order to contribute to my household's income, I went on GAU [general assistance/unemployable]. I knew GAU is a safety net for people like me, who are unable to work because of a disability. There was no shame when I went to the window to sign up, as I had no choice but to ask for help. I found that early morning was the best time to go to the welfare office, since there are fewer people. I was assigned a caseworker. There were forms to fill out, lines to stand in, chairs to wait in. But soon my check for three hundred and thirty-nine dollars came once a month, and it was welcomed. I also received a medical coupon with my GAU. I began calling it the 'golden coupon.' It allowed me to see doctors, and the state paid for it. Thankfully, it covered medications, too.

"A year later, I was still waiting for my Social Security hearing when I received a letter from the Washington State Department of Social and Health Services, telling me that my benefits had been canceled because they had not received updated documentation. Even though this was just a computer error, it served as a reminder that I had no control over my life or my finances.

"It took eighteen months to finally get my Social Security disability benefits," Betty says. "Due to another computer error, I received my first disability check months after I was awarded benefits. It became a daily ritual to wait for the mail every afternoon and walk out to the mailbox, only to find it full of bills. It seemed very sad to me that society values a person who has a job more than a person who has become ill through no fault of her own and cannot work."

Andrew M. had a better experience in applying for disability ben-

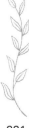

efits than most people we interviewed. "I had a great job and I was able to support myself," Andrew says. "Since I got diagnosed, I haven't been able to work. I've led an existence of not having enough money to support myself and having to live with family and friends. I finally applied for Social Security disability benefits when I realized that the FM wasn't going to go away. That was after four years of being sick. I was told that applying for disability was a long process and you get turned down the first few times just because, and finally the third time you end up going before a judge who makes the decision.

"But when I applied, mine went right through in two months, and I got an approval the first time around," he says. "But the diagnosis leading up to my disability is primarily based on depression and secondarily based on FM. They could award benefits based on a dual diagnosis, but they couldn't make a determination based on FM by itself."

Karin L. wasn't as lucky as Andrew. "At the time, I had been sick for less than six months. My mom suggested it and got the forms for me, thinking, 'If it lasts, you will at least have started the paperwork,'" Karin says. "So I filled them out and sent them in. I was of course denied the first time around, and the second time around I just didn't have the energy to deal with the paperwork and getting the letters from doctors to support my case. So I handed it over to my mom, who took one look and decided she didn't want to deal with it either. She called her lawyer. I think that may be the main reason I was approved at that time. The person who reviewed my case knew there was a lawyer involved and that we were serious about this because the lawyer had written to him to get a copy of everything in my file. My attorney wrote to other doctors requesting letters to support my case.

"It took about ten months from the time I initially applied until the time I was officially notified I was eligible for benefits. At that point, I found out I was not eligible for regular benefits because I was only twenty-three years old. I didn't have enough work credits to qualify for regular benefits. At that point, I learned that if you have received any money from any other source during the application process, it counts against you for getting Social Security, so I only received about eight hundred dollars in back benefits, rather than the several thousand I had anticipated. Ouch. I'm perfectly capable of handling money and being financially responsible, but I feel that I'm treated like I can't handle even the little bit of money Social Security will give you. I'm also receiving Section 8 rental assistance, so I finally have my own place.

"I still have a lot of anger towards Social Security and housing authorities," Karin says. "Because I'm on a very low income, I'm dependent on all these programs for help. I have four caseworkers. It's so complicated and ridiculous, it's amazing. And time-consuming, and tiring. It's frustrating because sometimes I feel like I know more about what they're supposed to be doing than they do. One thing I'm learning is that frustration really exhausts me. I beat on pillows, scream in the car. I feel like Big Brother is watching me. I feel like everything I do, I have to report or tell someone. I feel like I cannot make decisions about how much of my income I am willing to spend on rent versus other things."

Karin has been receiving disability benefits for about six years now. "I'm glad it's there," she says, "because I would be up a creek without it. I would not be able to afford to live on my own. I don't like the way the system is set up. I don't think it's very supportive or very 'health-giving,' for lack of a better term. The amount of energy and effort I expend dealing with Social Security and other agencies is enormous, ridiculous, and way out of proportion to the amount of money I'm getting from them. Some days I feel that my full-time job is not to go out and work, but to deal with agencies."

FM and CFS patients must actively defend their rights against the health insurance companies, private insurance companies, Social Security, and the court system that would deny their claims of disability. Education and knowledge are your best tools in fighting the system. The fact that you are successful in the face of adversity helps everyone in this situation. We thank the people who went before us, as their courage and perseverance made it a little easier for us to be taken seriously when applying for disability benefits.

223

■ Protecting Your Legal Rights

Morris Rosenberg

Morris Rosenberg, Esq., has practiced law in Seattle since 1975. He is a graduate of the University of Virginia School of Law. Mr. Rosenberg has been special district counsel for the Washington State Bar Association since 1984. In that capacity, he investigates and makes recommendations regarding complaints of misconduct against attorneys. Mr. Rosenberg limits his practice to the representation of injured people, employment discrimination, and family-law cases.

My law firm handles mostly personal injury cases. We represent people who were injured at the fault of someone else. I have noticed some trends that might explain why it is so difficult for an injured person to receive a fair resolution of claims where FM and CFS are involved. I think it primarily goes back to the fact that insurance companies exist to make a profit. Insurance companies take in premium dollars, and their goal is to pay out the smallest amounts they can, because that's obviously the way their profits stay large or increase. FM is a big controversy even within the medical community itself, which gives insurance carriers a fair amount of ammunition. They exploit that controversy to their advantage.

However, the legal system is getting more sophisticated. FM cases are becoming a battle of experts; typically, hired experts who charge high "witness fees" to be involved in a case. One would have no trouble finding an expert with good credentials on virtually any side of any issue. Insurance companies tend to react with skepticism to the assertion that the injured party has FM—because adjusters want juries to believe that people are just out to make a lot of money. Insurance adjusters (and some medical doctors and health-care providers as well) believe that people are simply looking for money and then make amazing recoveries once their cases are settled. There are some studies around, mostly in England, that indicate that settlement of a case has little, if anything, to do with the long-term symptomatology and how people fare. Once the case is settled, the pain remains.

In the cases I handle, which are mostly motor vehicle accidents, the individual often has a history of some medical problems; maybe they've been treated for depression, maybe they've seen a variety of doctors and complained of somewhat nondescript symptoms. These situations are exploited by insurance companies. They do all they can to make juries believe that the medical difficulties predated the accident. I have had several cases in which a person had a very clean medical history prior to the motor vehicle accident (or the trauma that the treating doctors indicate is the cause of the FM); those cases tend to go better for the injured person. When the onset of symptoms can be more clearly traced to a physical trauma, the injured party will generally receive a higher settlement or award.

I now have a case in which my client's own insurance company wants her to be examined by someone who doesn't even believe that FM exists. It certainly is indicative to me that it's not accepted by the insurance industry any more than it was ten years ago. I think as the general public gets more educated, we will find that there is quite a high incidence of FM. Perhaps it will get more accepted by the insurance industry, but I think it's an uphill battle.

Why do insurance companies tend to offer such small and modest amounts in these situations? Because of the existing controversy within the medical community, insurance companies have a lot of success in cases that go all the way to trial, with the juries awarding modest awards. The other difficulty in litigating cases involving FM is the fact that the insurance company has a right to have the client examined by doctors of their choice, and of course they want to send the patient to a doctor who does not believe that FM exists. And there is no shortage of physicians in the medical community with that attitude. Making my client go to such a doctor does not constitute an "independent exam" if the doctor is predisposed to think FM does not exist.

The situation I often see is one in which a person is injured in a modest auto accident and presents with modest soft-tissue damage and whiplash. Over the next four or five months, instead of improving, the injured person gets worse and gets frustrated, so they look for another doctor or different kind of care. Then the client has established a history of going to several doctors, not because they're looking for one to help them pull off a scam, but because they're simply not getting any better. Insurance companies will say that person is just trying to work the system and make it look like they've needed a lot of care to get better. They'll say the person is running up big medical bills in an effort to convince a jury or an insurance company that they have a lot of pain as a result of that low-impact auto accident.

With FM, this kind of history is very typical, because if you don't get into the right stream of care, you're not going to get the diagnosis. So it's common for me to get people who have gone to the emergency room, were told to wear a cervical collar for a while, and have maybe taken some nonsteroidal anti-inflammatories. They try that for a while, they don't get better, so they go to their family physician, then maybe to an orthopedist, who refers them to physical therapy. That doesn't help either, so they look for something else. They go to chiropractic care, and if that doesn't work, then they'll go somewhere else. They'll have to find a fairly sophisticated physician or somebody who will refer them to a rheumatologist. This doctor will take a good and detailed history, which is critical, and finally come up with the diagnosis.

Generally, few cases go all the way to trial. One of my cases was settled literally on the courthouse steps the day before the trial was to begin. That case was set to go to trial in Oregon in a county where the highest FM award from a jury was just over a hundred thousand dollars. There was a case in British Columbia a few years ago where the person was awarded almost seven hundred thousand dollars. The best FM case I had from the standpoint of dollar recovery was just under two hundred thousand dollars.

In any event, insurance companies know that they can find experts and doctors who will put some other diagnosis on it, like chronic depression. The person is then "crazy until proven otherwise." I've heard that term at several conferences I've attended, and people with FM run into that kind of attitude with insurance adjusters. I find that jury verdicts tend to be fairly modest in general with reference to "soft tissue injury," where the injury is typically to the musculature or the ligaments or tendons, with no broken bones or noticeable scarring. People look okay. Most of my clients, if not all of them, who have FM certainly look okay. Jurors have trouble awarding large sums of money in those situations. I think that plaintiffs' lawyers are having increasing difficulty in getting fair awards for their clients.

One client of mine had no prior history of any type of aches, pains, difficulty sleeping, or headaches. She was very healthy. She was a passenger in a car that was hit at fifty miles an hour. The vehicle did suffer a lot of physical damage, even though a collision can be low-impact and still trigger FM. My client ultimately dropped out of school and almost became a recluse: financially dependent upon a fiancé, with all the classic symptoms of FM. The insurance company sent her to an orthopedist; FM is not an orthopedic injury, but they sent her to an orthopedist anyway. They also had her see a psychiatrist for a psychiatric evaluation. And it was that hired psychiatrist's opinion that her problems were related not to the accident but to events that occurred when she was fourteen years old—a psychological trauma for which she had had only one counseling session. So fifteen years later, that's what the insurance adjuster said caused all her problems. Under the circumstances, we got a good settlement, although for the injured person no amount of money is going to make their medical situation any better.

To some extent, I think the public has heard a lot of public relations "spin" from the insurance injury about their rates going up, about people getting paid a lot of money for nothing. Everyone has heard about the lady who spilled her coffee and sued McDonald's. Those rare cases always make the headlines. What does not make the headlines are people who are legitimately injured; they have had significant impact on their lives, but they get little or no award. Those stories are not particularly newsworthy, but they're much more common than runaway jury awards are. In most states, if you sue because you can't settle your claim, you sue the person who caused the accident, not their insurance company. But in any event, either party has a constitutional right to a jury trial, and typically the insurance company will then demand a jury trial because they know they generally can do better in front of a jury.

It is important to remember not to tell anyone at the accident site that you are not injured. It is very common for people who are legitimately injured not to feel the effects of the injuries until hours, days, or even months later. Telling a police officer or someone else at the scene that you are not injured can come back to haunt you. We have all had situations where we have had a strenuous athletic workout and do not feel sore or achy until the next day. This can easily be the situation in an automobile accident, where there may be injuries to muscles, tendons, and ligaments not visible to the naked eye. If there is any chance you may be injured, have yourself checked out by a qualified physician at the first opportunity.

If you are injured in a car accident, I urge you to at least talk to an attorney who is experienced in personal injury law. Almost all lawyers who practice in that arena will meet initially with the person at no charge to discuss their legal rights. Most are also candid enough to tell you whether it makes sense to hire an attorney. Regrettably, insurance companies will use every means they can to limit their liability. Insurance companies are adept at finding an "expert" who can be paid to say anything in support of the insurance company. Be wary of insurance company representatives who advise you not to seek an attorney, or who try to talk you into signing their medical records release forms. This is in their best interest, not yours.

▨ A Patient's Story: Hilary S.

Hilary is twenty-nine years old and lives in Seattle with her husband. She is now a successful real-estate agent.

I was a passenger in a three-car collision in December 1993 in New York. We were rear-ended. I was immediately injured: my neck and my right arm hurt from bracing against the crash. The police wrote on the accident report that I was injured. We went to the hospital immediately; they diagnosed whiplash, neck sprain, and muscle strain.

I was twenty-three years old at the time. I thought I would just go to the chiropractor for a while and eventually recover. I had been seeing a chiropractor prior to the accident due to another car accident several years earlier. I had some minor back problems from that and from being a dancer at an early age. I went through two medical exams (at the request of the insurance company) and passed them both, but the doctors felt I still needed medical treatment. The insurance company paid all of my medical bills related to the car accident. Unfortunately, I was slowly getting worse. At the time of the accident, I had been actively looking for work and thinking about getting a master's degree.

I decided to move to Seattle to continue my job search there. When I finally found a job, I just couldn't do the work. I suddenly became very tired, irritable, and forgetful, and I was constantly in pain. I wasn't sure what was happening to me. I didn't correlate any of my symptoms to one condition. I thought my pain was due solely to the car accident, and the fatigue was from working long hours in a stressful job. I attributed the forgetfulness to being preoccupied. My sleeping patterns changed; it didn't matter how long I had slept the night before. I always felt tired.

At this point, I had no idea that something was seriously wrong with me. I hired an attorney in Seattle to handle my case in New York. The attorney encouraged me to go to an injury rehabilitation doctor he knew. I started seeing him in November 1994. I was in his clinic three or four times a week doing massage, biofeedback, TENS therapy, and lifting weights. Every time I picked up so much as a three-pound weight, I felt so much pain. Sometimes I got this pain in my head that hurt so badly I thought I had a brain tumor and was going to die. It was probably a migraine. I couldn't exercise without having pain. The doctor would say to me, "No pain, no gain." He said, "When you are done here, you will be one hundred percent recovered." He never listened to my complaints. I was so sick. Three months later, I was worse off than when I started. I was probably in treatment ten hours a week. The cost all ended up on lien, because my insurance company didn't recognize the fact that FM was related to the car accident. They cut my benefits off.

When I was first diagnosed, I felt relieved that there was actually a name to explain what was going on. I had a major decision to make: Do I quit work, go on welfare, file for Social Security disability, or do I continue working and suffering, and end up hospitalized? My choice was bittersweet. I chose to stop working because my health means more to me than anything. If you don't have your health, you have nothing. I thought, "I'm young, I got diagnosed right before my twenty-fifth birthday, and I will get better and get right back to work." I am a very ambitious and motivated person, so I told myself, "I can get past this." Little did I know what kind of journey I was about to go through.

I became frightened and full of humility. I couldn't believe this was happening to me. No one in my family has ever been on welfare. My family couldn't help me financially. My parents are divorced and my father didn't help me at all. I was living on three hundred and thirty-nine dollars a month and one hundred and twenty dollars in food stamps. At the time, I was living with my boyfriend; he moved with me to Seattle, and he was working to help supplement the bills, but it was really frightening. I had to use my credit card to pay for emergency bills. I would go to food banks when the food stamps ran out. I felt like I was going farther into the ground. I was ill, poor, and unable to work. I had more stress during those months than at any other time in my life. I learned so much about survival in a manner that I never thought I would experience. People treated me differently because I was on welfare. It was awful.

The first portion of my settlement came in March 1996. We had mediation against the insurance company of the driver in the second car. And then the rest was settled in October 1996. I feel very fortunate that I got some type of compensation. It certainly made things a little easier. I have paid around fifty thousand dollars out of pocket for medical bills to date. The settlement money was put into a special needs irrevocable trust. My mother is the trustee. It allowed me to stay on state and federal "needy" programs without penalty. The trust can only pay for things that are not paid for by any other means. The trust cannot give me personal income. An attorney set this up for me.

I am feeling a lot better, although I don't feel 100 percent well. Obviously, I didn't ever expect that I would be disabled. I think it has changed me for the better. I think people take their lives for granted when everything comes so easily or there's no tragedy in their life. Time is so much more valuable to me than it once was. One minute I'm healthy, the next minute a seventy-three-year old man hits me, and the next minute I'm bedridden and sick. Someone once said to me, "If you live in the moment, you heal the past and create the future." That's where I'm trying to be now, healing the past and creating the future.

■ ■ ■

That's it for us. Now here are a few pages to record your personal story, comments, and feedback. We would like to receive your stories and suggestions for possible inclusion in a future update of this book. Please send them by email to

fmcfsbook@earthlink.net or home.earthlink.net\~fmcfsbook

with a copy to hhi@hunterhouse.com. Or you can send them by U.S. mail (typewritten, please) to Mari Skelly, c/o Hunter House Publishers, P.O. Box 2914, Alameda CA 94501-0914.

We are tentatively planning to produce a stretching and exercise video specifically for people with chronic pain, so let us know if you are interested!

■ A Patient's Story: _____
(your name here)

233

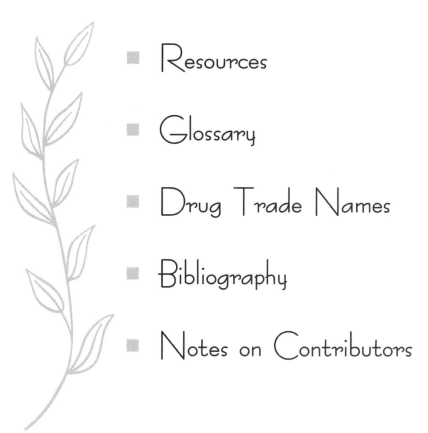

■ Resources

■ Glossary

■ Drug Trade Names

■ Bibliography

■ Notes on Contributors

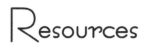

Resources

Alternative Treatment Web Sites

http://www.amerchiro.org   Provides information on chiropractic licensing, accreditation, education, and research articles, plus a list of members.

http://www.amtamassage.org   Includes an explanation of massage therapists' credential issues and what qualities to look for in a massage therapist.

http://www.healthy.net   Homepage of Health World, a comprehensive, global network that integrates alternative and conventional health information; pages include MedLine and the Marketplace. Site also provides information on Health World's speakers' network and offers a bookstore search.

http://www.homeopathic.org   Homepage of the National Center for Homeopathy. Provides state-by-state listing of homeopathic practitioners and information.

http://www.institute-dc.org   Homepage of the Cost Containment Research Institute, which offers a free thirty-two-page booklet with information on largely unknown programs through which many pharmaceutical companies offer free or discounted prescription drugs. The booklet discusses free and low-cost prescription drugs available to patients who are referred by physicians and who meet eligibility requirements, and it also contains contact information for five discount mail-order services.

http://www.medicalacupuncture.org   Provides acupuncture information, medical references with links to other sites, and a practitioner list.

http://www.naturopathic.org   Provides practitioner lists, state organizations, and licensing and credential explanations from the American Association of Naturopathic Physicians.

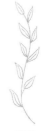

http://www.rxlist.com   Provides a comprehensive listing of drug names and indications.

237

Additional Web Sites

http://www.cdc.gov   U.S. Centers for Disease Control and Prevention

http://www.geocities.com/HotSprings/Spa/5252   Guaifenesin support group

http://www.ncbi.nlm.nih.gov/pubmed   Free online information service through the U.S. National Library of Medicine

http://www.niaid.nih.gov   National Institute of Allergy and Infectious Diseases

Newsletters

CFIDS Chronicle
Published by the CFIDS Association of America
P.O. Box 220398, Charlotte NC 28222-0398   Tel. (704) 365-2343

Fibromyalgia Network
P.O. Box 31750, Tucson AZ 85751-1750   Tel. (800) 853-2929

The Fibromyalgia Times
Published by the FM Alliance of America
P.O. Box 21990, Columbus OH 43221-0990   Tel. (614) 457-4222

Fibromyalgia Health Letter
Published by the Arthritis Foundation
P.O. Box 921907, Norcross GA 30010-1907   Tel. (404) 872-7100
Medical questions for the *Wellness Letter* can be sent to:
"Ask the Experts", 1330 West Peachtree Street, Atlanta GA 30309
                                          email: fwlmail@arthritis.org

Healthwatch
Published by Pro Health, Inc.
1187 Coast Village Road, #1-280, Santa Barbara CA 93108-2794
                                          Tel. (800) 366-6056

INFA News
Published by the Inland Northwest Fibromyalgia Association
933 West Third, Suite 211, Spokane WA 99201   Tel. (509) 838-3001

Health Points
Published by To Your Health, Inc.
17007 East Colony Drive, #105, Fountain Hills AZ 85268
Tel. (800) 801-1406

Organizations

Acupuncture Association of Washington
P.O. Box 31385, Seattle WA 98103   Tel. (206) 329-9094

American Association for Chronic Fatigue Syndrome
c/o Harborview Medical Center
325 Ninth Avenue, Box 359780, Seattle WA 98104   Tel. (206) 521-1932
Fax (206) 521-1930
Web site: http://www.aacfs.org   email: aacfs@aacfs.org

Arthritis Foundation
P.O. Box 921907, Norcross GA 30010-9904   Tel. (404) 872-7100
Question-and-answer line (800) 283-7800
Web site: http://www.arthritis.org

CFIDS Association of America
P.O. Box 220398, Charlotte NC 28222-0398   Tel. (800) 442-3437

Center for Fatigue Sciences
28240 Agoura Road, Suite 201, Agoura Hills CA 91301
Tel. (818) 991-9800

Chemical Injury Information Network
P.O. Box 301, White Sulphur Springs MT 59645   Tel. (406) 547-2255

Wisconsin Viral Research Group
10437 Innovation Drive, Suite 321, Milwaukee WI 53226
Tel. (414) 774-0311

National CFIDS Foundation
103 Aletha Road, Needham MA 02492   Tel. (781) 449-3535
Web site: http://www.cfidsfoundation.org

National Fibromyalgia Research Association
P.O. Box 500, Salem OR 97308 (Provides a patient information packet)

239

Optimum Health Institute of San Diego
6970 Central Avenue, Lemongrove CA 91945   Tel. (619) 464-3346
Fax (619) 589-4098   Web site: http://www.optimumhealth.org

Social Security Administration
Office of Disability, Professional Relations Branch
3-A-10 Operations, 6401 Security Boulevard, Baltimore MD 21235
Tel. (800) 772-1213   Claims (800) 431-2804

Social Security Disability Advocates
23930 Michigan Avenue, Dearborn MI 48124   Tel. (800) 628-2887

Washington Intractable/Chronic Pain Advocacy
P.O. Box 10019, Spokane WA 99209-0019   Tel. (509) 328-8534

Wilson's Syndrome Foundation
P.O. Box 539, Summerfield FL 34492   Tel. (800) 621-7006
          Web site: http://www.wilsonssyndrome.com

Support Groups

Call the Arthritis Foundation at (404) 872-7100 (toll-free Q&A line
[800] 283-7800) for a list of support groups in your area.

Products and Supplements

Alpha Stim Units
Nancy Campbell
Distributor, Therapeutic Resources
P.O. Box 12608, Mill Creek WA 98082-0608   Tel. (425) 745-8505
          (800) FOR-PAIN
          Web site: http://www.painsolutions.com

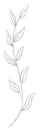

The Alpha Stim 100 is classified as a combination transcutaneous electrical nerve stimulator (TENS) and a cranial electrotherapy stimulator (CES). Broadly classified as a TENS unit, Alpha Stim 100 microcurrent electrotherapy works by using tiny currents similar in type and amount to the electricity that naturally occurs in the body. For some people, Alpha Stim effectively helps to manage sleep, pain, and anxiety. It has also been used successfully on people in drug rehabilitation. No significant side effects have been reported in more than 100 human research studies.

CFIDS & FM Health Resource

1187 Coast Village Road, Suite 1-280, Santa Barbara CA 93108-2794

Tel. (800) 366-6056   Web site: http://www.immunesupport.com

This patient-owned organization sells herbal/vitamin supplements through its newsletter and via the Internet, then donates its profits to CFS research. More than two million dollars has been donated to date. Services also include *Healthwatch Online,* the largest CFS and FM online newsletter in the country, as well as a scientific abstract library and an online feature, *Ask Immune Support,* which enables the user to submit personal health questions.

Metagenics

Web site: http://www.ultrabalance.com

UltraClear Sustain, produced by Metagenics, is a gastrointestinal nutritional supplement only available through licensed health-care providers. To find a distributor in the United States, call (800) 692-9400. To find a distributor outside the United States, call Healthcom at (800) 843-9660 or access the Web site listed above.

Treatment Providers

Contact information for the treatment providers who contributed to this book can be found in the Notes on Contributors section.

Bastyr University Natural Health Clinic

1307 North 45th Street, Seattle WA 98103   Tel. (206) 632-0354

Dr. Robyn DeSautel

DeSautel Chiropractic

5902 California Avenue SW, Seattle WA 98136   Tel. (206) 932-3718

Dynamics of Physical Development Consultants (Geoff Gluckman)

1840 41st Avenue, #102-141, Capitola CA 95010   Tel. (831) 685-8211
                                                                              (800) 7-SEMINAR

Web site: http://www.dpdc-mbf.com email: gluckmanfeat@dpdc-mbf.com Call the toll-free number to obtain a CD-ROM; access the Web site to obtain a list of Muscle Balance and Function Development classes in your area.

241

Glossary

acupuncture A diagnostic system used to treat illness, manage chronic disorders, and alleviate pain. Part of traditional Chinese medicine, it promotes health through prevention and maintenance, encourages healing, and improves functioning. (Chinese medicine, the most widely used healing system in the world, combines acupuncture, herbs, cupping, moxabustion [burning the herb moxa to add heat to the body], massage, diet, and gentle exercise to correct energy imbalances in the body.) Acupuncture involves the insertion of needles (sometimes combined with the application of heat or electrical stimulation) at precise points on the body.

acute A disease or condition with a rapid onset and a short, severe course.

aerobic exercise "Aerobic" means "in the presence of oxygen." Any exercise during which the energy needed is supplied by the oxygen inspired. Aerobic exercise is required for sustained periods of hard work and vigorous athletic activity. Sustained aerobic activity stimulates and strengthens the heart and lungs, which improves the body's ability to deliver and utilize oxygen.

Alexander Technique A movement therapy that teaches students about improved use of the body and helps to identify and change poor or inefficient physical habits that may cause stress or fatigue. This system of physical retraining uses a series of simple movements that put the body into a state of balance and relaxation and encourages students to develop awareness and control in their daily activities. The Alexander Technique is the basis for some other movement techniques, such as Feldenkrais (see below).

arthritis Inflammation of a joint, which may cause swelling, redness, and pain. It is part of the category of rheumatic disease, in which there is an inflammatory condition involving the joints. (The broader term "rheumatic disease" refers to conditions in which there are changes in connective tissues, including muscle, tendons, joints, bursae, and fibrous tissues.) The two main types of arthritis are rheumatoid, an autoimmune disease, and osteoarthritis, also called degenerative joint disease.

autoimmune disease A disorder associated with the body's production of antibodies directed against its own tissues. It can be organ specific, such as Hashimoto's disease (which affects the thyroid), or systemic, such as systemic lupus erythematosus. Rheumatoid arthritis is an autoimmune disease.

biofeedback A system that trains the mind to gain voluntary control over autonomic body functions. Its goal is to help the patient use enhanced muscle awareness to develop better muscle utilization and release skills.

candida A complex medical syndrome caused by chronic overgrowth of the yeast Candida albicans in body tissues. General symptoms include chronic fatigue, loss of energy, general malaise, and decreased libido. Symptoms may be similar to those of FM and CFS. Most affected are the body's gastrointestinal system (bloating, gas, intestinal cramps, rectal itching, and altered bowel function), endocrine system (primarily menstrual complaints), nervous system (depression, irritability, and inability to concentrate), and immune system (allergies, chemical sensitivities, and low immune function). Treatment includes a low-carbohydrate diet, lactobacillus acidophilus (to promote normal floral growth in the gut), and antifungal medications. Major causes include use of antibiotics, birth control pills, steroids, or immune-suppressing drugs.

carpal tunnel syndrome A symptom complex resulting from compression of the median nerve in the wrist's carpal tunnel that results in pain, burning, tingling, or numbness in the fingers and hands. Pain sometimes extends to the elbow; the syndrome is frequently caused by repetitive stress.

chi The vital life energy that Asian medicine believes flows through the body's acupuncture meridians; known as *qi* in Japanese acupuncture and *prana* in Ayurvedic medicine.

chi kung A Chinese system of specific exercises designed to build *chi* and restore health.

Chinese medicine A system of medical treatment, thought, and practice developed over two millennia; its therapeutics include acupuncture, herbs, nutrition, massage, and movement techniques such as *tai chi* and *chi kung*.

chiropractic A health-care system that deals with the relationship between the spinal column and the nervous system. Its philosophy teaches that

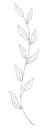

243

nerve impulses must flow in an unobstructed manner from the spinal nerves to all parts of the body in order for a person to enjoy harmony, vitality, and good health. It is the most widespread drugless, nonsurgical health system in the Western world.

chronic Of long duration; used to describe a disease or condition that progresses slowly and lasts more than six months.

chronic fatigue syndrome (CFS) A specific illness characterized by severe, persistent fatigue, often associated with difficulties of sleep and concentration, aching muscles and joints, headaches, sore throat, and depression. In clinical populations, it is most commonly diagnosed in previously healthy women between the ages of twenty and fifty, but it can afflict people of all ages and socioeconomic groups throughout the world.

cognition Awareness and perception of reality, including all aspects of perceiving, thinking, and remembering.

cognitive behavioral modification A psychotherapeutic technique that uses guided self-discovery, imaging, self-instruction, and related forms of elicited cognition as the principal mode of treatment.

craniosacral therapy A gentle, noninvasive, hands-on manipulative technique that helps to detect and correct imbalances in the body's craniosacral system, which can cause various sensory, motor, or intellectual dysfunctions. The body's craniosacral system is comprised of the brain, spinal cord, cerebrospinal fluid, cranial dural membrane, cranial bones, and sacrum. This therapy is used by many health-care practitioners, including medical doctors, dentists, chiropractors, osteopaths, naturopaths, acupuncturists, and licensed body workers.

debilitating Leading to limited ability; causing a loss of strength or energy.

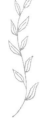

dermatomyocytis A rare autoimmune disease in which there is inflammation of the skin and subcutaneous tissue and necrosis (death) of the muscle fibers. Symptoms include fever, weight loss, skin lesions, and aching muscles. As the disease progresses, use of the arms and legs may be lost. Only one person in 300,000 has this illness. Treatment includes steroids.

diagnosis The act or process of identifying or determining the nature or cause of a disease or injury through evaluation of patient history and examination and review of laboratory data; also refers to the opinion that results from such evaluation.

Eastern medicine A term used to refer to non-Western systems of medicine. See also acupuncture and Chinese medicine.

elimination diet A naturopathic treatment for food allergies in which the patient avoids allergic foods in order to return to a state of health. It generally takes three to five days for the intestinal tract to eliminate all the offending food in the body. The patient then slowly reintroduces each allergic food to see if the body reacts. If it does, avoidance is recommended.

Feldenkrais method A movement technique focused on body/mind integration that uses movement to enhance communication between the brain and body. Lessons, either one-on-one or in a group, seek to improve people's awareness along with their physical and mental performance. The practitioner guides the student through a series of precise movements that alter habitual patterns and provide new learning directly to the neuromuscular system. Lessons are usually done on a padded table with the student fully clothed.

fibromyalgia (FM) According to the American College of Rheumatology, FM is a condition diagnosed by a history of chronic, generalized aching and the finding, upon physical exam, of at least eleven out of eighteen "tender points" (see below). These sites are more tender than other points in the body.

growth hormone A substance that stimulates growth and body tissues; specifically, a secretion of the anterior lobe of the pituitary gland that directly influences protein, carbohydrate, and lipid metabolism and controls the rate of skeletal and visceral growth.

Hashimoto's disease An autoimmune disorder of the thyroid gland in which antibodies are produced against thyroid tissues; most common in middle-aged women. Treatment is administration of thyroid hormones (see also hypothyroidism).

heal To restore to health, balance, or soundness; to cure.

holistic medicine A form of therapy aimed at treating the whole person, not just the body part or parts in which a symptom occurs; the term refers to the whole body or to the body/mind/spirit connection.

homeopathic/homeopathy A system of medicine based on the concept that "like cures like." Its basic premise is that any substance that is capable of producing symptoms in a healthy person can cure those symptoms in a sick person. Homeopathic remedies are diluted agents or substances that assist the body in utilizing its own energy to regain balance and health, and are derived from a variety of plant, mineral, and chemical substances. Homeopathic treatment addresses the patient's entire body and personality and does not focus solely upon the patient's specific disease or symptom.

hyperthyroidism A condition of excessive functional activity of the thyroid gland. It occurs most commonly as part of a syndrome that may include enlarged thyroid (goiter) and abnormal protrusion of the eyes (exophthalmia). Also known as Graves' disease.

hypnotherapy A therapy using hypnosis; especially useful for management of chronic pain.

hypothyroidism A deficiency of thyroid gland activity with underproduction of the hormone thyroxine. In its severe form, it is called myxedema and is characterized by physical and mental sluggishness, loss of hair, weight gain, cold intolerance, skin coarsening, mental dulling, fatigue, and menstrual irregularities. Treatment is administration of thyroid hormones.

irritable bladder syndrome Also known as interstitial cystitis; increased frequency of contractions in the urinary bladder, associated with an increased need to urinate.

irritable bowel syndrome A group of symptoms that comprises the most common disorder presented by patients seeking a gastroenterologist. Symptoms include altered bowel habits, with diarrhea, constipation, or both; abdominal pain, gas, and bloating; and an absence of any other detectable organic disease. It is frequently treated with a high-fiber diet and Bentyl, an antispasmodic, for pain.

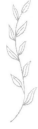

246

Lyme disease An infection caused by a spiral-shaped bacterium called

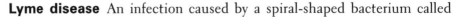

Borrelia burgdorferi, which is most commonly transmitted by the deer tick. A bulls-eye rash, with a round ring and central clearing, is the hallmark of Lyme disease. Several weeks after a bite from an infected tick, a person usually experiences flulike symptoms such as aches and pains in the muscles and joints, low-grade fever, or fatigue. Treatment includes antibiotics.

magnetic resonance imaging (MRI) A diagnostic test used by physicians to view the body's internal tissues and organs.

massage therapy The manipulation of soft tissue for therapeutic purposes, either by hand or with a mechanical or electrical apparatus. The use of touch to soothe or gain some degree of relief from pain is a universal human technique. Specific techniques include myofascial release therapy, Swedish massage, Rolfing, Hellerwork, and movement-based techniques such as the Feldenkrais method and Alexander Technique.

multiple chemical sensitivity (MCS) A term that, like "environmental illness," describes states of ill health caused by exposure to substances normally present in the environment, including foods, molds, pollens, and dusts, as well as chemicals, that do not normally make otherwise healthy people ill. The affected person becomes hypersensitized to these substances, causing the immune system to overreact. MCS symptoms can affect any bodily system and may include headaches, nausea, fatigue, dizziness, confusion, muscle weakness, depression, anxiety, and many other physical and emotional reactions.

Muscle Balance and Function Development (MBF) A system focused on postural realignment that applies a progression of properly sequenced, individualized exercises to restore function to the body. The program's evaluation process reveals muscular imbalances that cause postural misalignment, compensated motion, and injury.

myofascial release therapy The prefix myo- means muscle. Myofascial release is a hands-on technique used by therapists to relieve soft tissue (muscle) from the grip of abnormally tight fascia (connective tissue). It is a mild and gentle form of stretching that is used to relieve pain and improve physical function.

naturopathic medicine A system of holistic and nontoxic approaches to medical therapy, with a strong emphasis on disease prevention and wellness optimization. A licensed naturopathic physician attends a four-year, graduate-level naturopathic medical school and is educated in all the same basic sciences as a medical doctor while also studying naturopathic techniques. Therapeutics include clinical nutrition, acupuncture, homeopathic medicine, botanical medicine, psychology, and lifestyle counseling.

neuralgia Pain in a nerve or along the course of one or more nerves. It is caused by inflammation of or injury to a nerve or group of nerves and is usually a sharp, spasmlike pain that may occur at intervals.

neurohormones Hormones that stimulate the neural (nervous) system.

neurology The branch of health science that deals with the nervous system, both normal and diseased. A neurologist is a specialist in the treatment of neurological diseases.

neurotransmitters Substances that are released from a neuron and travel along the neuron path to either excite (turn on) or inhibit (turn off) a target cell in the central nervous system (see also serotonin and Substance P). These substances modify or transmit nerve impulses.

nutrition The process by which a living organism assimilates food and uses it for growth, liberation of energy, and replacement of lost cells. The stages include mastication, digestion, absorption, assimilation, and excretion. Nutrition is the science or study that deals with human food and nourishment. A nutritionist is a specialist in the study and application of nutrition theory.

objective criteria In the context of diagnosis, these are medical testing methods (such as X-rays, urinalysis, and blood sample testing) that can detect the presence of illness or establish a diagnosis (see also subjective criteria).

opioids Opioids are drugs that mimic the activity of opiate drugs, which are named after their natural source, the opium poppy. The poppy contains several active chemicals, including the opiates morphine and codeine. Synthetically produced opioids include meperidine and methadone. These drugs bind to opiate receptors in the central nervous system and spur the release of endorphins, painkillers, and encephalins, the body's natural opiates.

osteopathy A system of medicine based on the theory that disturbances in the musculoskeletal system affect other body parts and can cause

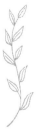

many disorders that can be corrected by various hands-on manipulative techniques used in conjunction with conventional therapeutic procedures. A doctor of osteopathy specializes in, among other things, the use of osteopathic manipulation.

pain management specialist A physician who specializes in treating chronic pain conditions.

physical therapy An exercise system aimed at helping the patient avoid abnormal movement patterns and returning them to the highest possible level of function. A physical therapist treats physical dysfunction or injury by the use of therapeutic exercise and the application of modalities intended to restore or facilitate normal body function.

physiology All the functions of a living organism or any of its parts.

podiatry A specialized medical field dealing with the care and study of the foot, including its anatomy, pathology, and medical and surgical treatment. A podiatrist is a specialist in the treatment of foot disorders.

psychiatry A branch of medicine that seeks to treat mental and emotional disorders. A psychiatrist is a physician who specializes in the treatment of such disorders.

psychotherapy The treatment of mental and emotional disorders through the use of psychological techniques designed to encourage communication of conflicts and insight into problems, with the goals being personality growth and behavioral modification.

rheumatology The study and treatment of rheumatic diseases. Rheumatism is any of several pathological conditions of the muscles, tendons, joints, bones, or nerves that are characterized by discomfort and disability. Rheumatology is comprised of those conditions that tend to be chronic and involve the musculoskeletal system: joints, tendons, and muscles. Rheumatological conditions include both congenital and inflammatory arthritis; autoimmune diseases that affect joints, connective tissues, and other parts of the body, such as lupus, Sjogren's syndrome, and scleroderma; and conditions involving chronic pain and muscle pain. A rheumatologist specializes in treating these disorders. The training of a rheumatologist typically lasts two or more years beyond internal medicine training.

sciatica A sharp, spasmlike pain that occurs along the sciatic nerve; felt in the back and down the back of the thigh to the ankle. It is caused by inflammation of or injury to the sciatic nerve.

serotonin A hormone and neurotransmitter, 5-hydroxytryptamine (5-HT), that is found in many tissues, including blood platelets, intestinal mucosa, the pineal body, and the central nervous system. It has many functions in the body, including inhibition of gastric secretion, stimulation of smooth muscles, and vasoconstriction. Serotonin has been determined to play a key role in FM and CFS. Because many antidepressants function by modifying how serotonin is used in the body (especially in the central nervous system), they may be prescribed as part of the treatment of FM and CFS.

sleep apnea A sleep disorder characterized by respiratory interruptions during REM sleep (a stage of sleep characterized by rapid eye movement.) Symptoms include repeated nighttime awakening and excessive daytime sleepiness. It is commonly treated with medications and a continuous positive airway pressure (CPAP) machine, which keeps the body's airway open during sleep.

somatic Of, relating to, or affecting the physical body, especially as distinguished from the mind or the environment.

subjective criteria Symptoms such as pain or fatigue that are reported by the patient but cannot be confirmed by conventional objective diagnostic tools such as X-rays, blood analysis, etc. (see also objective criteria).

Substance P An irritative neurotransmitter present in nerve cells that are scattered throughout the body and in special endocrine cells in the gut; it increases the contractions of gastrointestinal smooth muscle and causes vasodilation. It is a sensory neurotransmitter involving pain, touch, and temperature. Studies indicate that FM patients have up to three times the normal amount of Substance P in their nerve cells.

syndrome A group of symptoms that collectively indicate or characterize a disease, psychological disorder, or other abnormal condition.

tai chi A Chinese system of physical exercises that is based on principles of rhythmic movement, equilibrium of body weight, and effortless breathing, designed to build *chi* (vital life energy). Originally developed as a martial art for self-defense, it is characterized by progressing slowly and continuously, without strain, through a sequence of contrasting movements. The objective is to achieve health and tranquillity through movement while developing the mind and body; it teaches students how to control the nervous system in order to put the entire body at rest.

temporomandibular joint disorder (TMJ) A dysfunction in which there is a clicking or grinding sensation in the temporomandibular joint; includes pain in or about the ears, tiredness, soreness of the jaw muscle upon waking, and stiffness of the jaw itself. Treatment may include both medical and dental intervention and trigger-point and tender-point injections (see below).

tender point A sensitive, painful area that is sore to the touch and found only in FM patients. There are eighteen such sites in the body; a diagnosis of FM is based upon the finding of at least eleven of these tender points on exam.

thyroid The largest of the endocrine glands, which produces hormones vital for maintaining normal growth and metabolism. The hormones it secretes are triodothyronine (T3) and tetraiodothyronine (T4). Its disorders include hyperthyroidism, hypothyroidism, Hashimoto's disease, and Wilson's Syndrome (see those glossary entries).

toxin A poison produced by some plants, animals, pathogenic bacteria, and human activities, such as burning fossil fuels or production of industrial wastes. Exposure to these substances can sometimes be fatal.

trigger point Differs from the tender points found in FM patients (see above). Part of a specific pain pattern found in myofascial pain syndrome, a trigger point is a hypersensitive area in the myofascia (muscle and connective tissue) that is very painful to the touch. Stimulation of this point also "refers" a sensation of pain to another part of the body.

trigger-point and tender-point injections The use of various techniques to sedate, desensitize, or eliminate trigger or tender points. By sedating pain in these points, the myofascia are allowed to relax and let the area normalize, which stops the referral of pain to other parts of the body. Anesthetics or saline may be injected, or a dry needle may be inserted.

vocational rehabilitation A program designed to aid a person in returning to functionality and employment after a chronic illness. Elements can include counseling, job training, education, and vocational retraining.

Western medicine The system of medicine practiced by most medical doctors in the United States and other parts of the Western world; also known as conventional medicine and allopathic medicine. It aims to produce relief through drugs, surgery, and other therapeutics.

Wilson's Syndrome A newly defined hypothyroid condition in which the body is unable to convert inactive hormone into active usable hormone. Treatment is with Cytomel, which contains liothyronine (T3).

yoga An Indian exercise and movement therapy designed to restore harmony, flexibility, and function to the body. Yoga purifies the body by releasing toxins and impurities. It works with the endocrine system and the nervous system and aligns the spine. It brings strength and stamina to the various muscle groups, and one of its most important benefits is that it aids the digestive system.

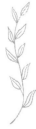

Drug Trade Names

The drugs listed below may be used to treat many conditions besides FM and CFS. However, the chart indicates how they are used specifically to treat FM and CFS.

Trade Name	Generic Name	Class/Indication
Ambien	zolpiden	sleeping aid
Bentyl	dicyclomine	antispasmodic
BuSpar	buspirone	sedative
Cytomel	liothyronine sodium	thyroid hormone
Deltasone	prednisone	anti-inflammatory
Desyrel	trazodone	antidepressant
Duragesic	fentanyl transdermal	narcotic analgesic patch
Elavil	amitriptyline	antidepressant
Endocet	oxycodone and acetaminophen	narcotic analgesic
Endodan	oxycodone and aspirin	narcotic analgesic
Flexeril	cyclobenzaprine	muscle relaxant
guaifenesin	guaifenesin	expectorant, removes waste matter from muscles
Imitrex	sumatriptan	migraine relief
Klonopin	clonazepam	benzodiazepine, antiseizure
Levsinex	hyoscyamine	antispasmodic
Lidocaine	lidocaine	local anesthetic, numbing agent
Lioresal	baclofen	muscle relaxant
methadone	methadone	narcotic analgesic
MS-Contin	morphine	narcotic analgesic
Motrin	ibuprofen	pain relief
Naprosyn	naproxen	NSAID
Neurontin	gabapentin	nerve pain reduction

Trade Name	Generic Name	Class/Indication
Norflex	orphenadrine citrate	muscle relaxant
Oxycontin	oxycodone	narcotic analgesic
Pamelor	nortriptyline	antidepressant
Paxil	paroxetine	antidepressant
Percocet	oxycodone and acetaminophen	narcotic analgesic
Percodan	oxycodone and aspirin	narcotic analgesic
Procaine	procaine	local anesthetic
Prozac	fluoxetine	antidepressant
Rheumatrex dp	methotrexate	autoimmune disease treatment
Robaxin	methocarbamol	muscle relaxant
Roxicet	oxycodone and acetaminophen	narcotic analgesic
Roxicodone	oxycodone	narcotic analgesic
Roxiprin	oxycodone and aspirin	narcotic analgesic
Serzone	nefazodone	antidepressant
Sinemet	carbidopa-levodopa	antidyskinetic
Sinequan	doxepin	antidepressant
Soma	carisoprodol	muscle relaxant
Synthroid	levothyroxine sodium	thyroid hormone
Toradol	Ketorolac	NSAID
Tranzene	clorazepate dipotassium	benzodiazepine, muscle relaxant
Tylenol 3	acetaminophen and codeine	narcotic analgesic
Tylox	oxycodone and acetaminophen	narcotic analgesic
Ultram	tramadol	opiate agonist/pain relief
Vicodin	hydrocodone/acetaminophen	narcotic analgesic
Voltaren	diclofenac	NSAID, pain relief
Wellbutrin	bupropion	antidepressant
Zoloft	sertraline	antidepressant

Bibliography

American Heritage Stedmen's Medical Dictionary. Boston, MA: Houghton Mifflin, 1995.

Anderson, Bob, and Jean E. Anderson. *Stretching.* Bolinas, CA: Shelter Publications, 1980.

Arthritis Foundation. *Your Personal Guide to Living Well with Fibromyalgia.* Atlanta, GA: Longstreet Press, 1997.

Barron's Dictionary of Medical Terms, 3rd edition. Hauppage, NY: Barron's Educational Series, 1994.

Beeken, Jenny. *Yoga of the Heart.* New York, NY: White Eagle Publishing Trust, 1990.

Borysenko, Joan, with Larry Rothstein. *Minding the Body, Mending the Mind.* New York: Addison-Wesley, 1987.

Bragg, Patricia, and Paul C. Bragg. *The Miracle of Fasting.* Santa Monica, CA: Health Science Press, 1997.

Brother Lawrence. *Practicing His Presence.* Translated by Frank C. Laubach and Gene Edwards. Augusta, ME: Christian Books Publishing House, 1988.

Castro, Miranda. *The Complete Homeopathy Handbook: A Guide to Everyday Health Care.* New York: St. Martin's Press, 1990.

Colbin, Annemarie. *Food and Healing.* New York: Ballantine Books, 1996.

Cousens, Gabriel. *Conscious Eating,* 2nd edition. Berkeley, CA: North Atlantic Books, 1999.

Foster, Richard J. *Celebration of Discipline: The Path to Spiritual Growth.* San Francisco, CA: HarperSanFrancisco, 1988.

Fransen, Jenny, and I. Jon Russell. *The Fibromyalgia Help Book: A Practical Guide to Living Better with Fibromyalgia.* St. Paul, MN: Smith House Press, 1996.

Fredericks, Carlton. *Arthritis: Don't Learn to Live with It.* New York: Perigee Books, 1981.

Gibson, Pamela Reed. "Environmental Illness/Multiple Chemical Sensitivities: Invisible Disabilities." In *Women with Disabilities: Found Voices,* edited by Lillian Holcomb and Mary E. Willmuth. Binghamton, NY: Haworth Press, 1993.

Gibson, Pamela Reed. *Multiple Chemical Sensitivity: A Survival Guide.* Oakland, CA: New Harbinger Publishers, 1999.

Griner, Thomas, and Maxine Nunes. *What's Really Wrong With You? A Revolutionary Look at How Muscles Affect Your Health.* Garden City Park, NY: Avery Publishing, 1996.

Hall, C., and L. Thein-Brody, eds. *Therapeutic Exercise: Moving Toward Function.* Philadelphia, PA: Lippincott, Williams & Wilkins, 1999.

Kabat-Zinn, Jon. *Full Catastrophe Living: Using the Wisdom of Your Body and Mind to Face Stress, Pain, and Illness.* New York: Dell Publishing, 1990.

Kaptchuk, Ted J. *The Web That Has No Weaver: Understanding Chinese Medicine.* New York: Congdon & Weed, 1993.

Kastner, Mark, and Hugh Burroughs. *Alternative Healing.* La Mesa, CA: Halcyon Publishing, 1993.

Kendall, Florence Peterson, Elizabeth Kendall McCreary, and Patricia Geise Provance. *Muscles Testing and Function.* Baltimore, MD: Williams & Wilkins, 1993.

Kushner, Harold. *When Bad Things Happen to Good People.* New York: Schocken Books, 1981.

Lorig, Kate, and J. Fries. *Arthritis Help Book,* 4th edition. New York: Addison-Wesley, 1995.

Lorig, Kate, et al. *Living a Healthy Life with Chronic Conditions.* Palo Alto, CA: Bull Publications, 1994.

Martinez, Martin. *Cannabis Indications: Scientific Aspects of Medical Marihuana.* Santa Rosa, CA: Lifevine Publications, 1998.

Martinson, Linda. *Poetry of Pain.* Lynnwood, WA: Simply Books, 1996. (Ordering information: P.O. Box 2205, Lynnwood, WA 98036-2205)

Melvin, Jeanne. *Fibromyalgia Syndrome: Getting Healthy.* American Occupational Therapy Association, 1996.

Miller-Keane Encyclopedia and Dictionary of Medicine, Nursing and Allied Health, 5th edition. Philadelphia, PA: W. B. Saunders Co., 1992.

Norberg, Tilda, and Robert D. Webber. *Stretch Out Your Hand: Exploring Healing Prayer.* Nashville, TN: Upper Room Publications, 1999.

Pellegrino, Dr. Mark J., M.D. *Fibromyalgia: Managing the Pain.* Columbus, OH: Anadem Publishing, 1993.

Penner, Barbara. *Managing Fibromyalgia: A Six-Week Course on Self-Care.* Meerkat Graphics Center, 1997. (Ordering information: Capital Physical Therapy Center, 25 South Ewing, Room 206, Helena, MT 59601, [406] 449-4066)

Pitchford, Paul. *Healing with Whole Foods: Oriental Traditions and Modern Nutrition.* Berkeley, CA: North Atlantic Books, 1996.

Pizzorono, Joseph, and Michael Murray, eds. *Encyclopedia of Natural Medicine,* 1st edition. Rocklin, CA: Prima Publishing, 1991.

Robbins, John, and Jia Patton. *May All Be Fed: A Diet for a New World.* New York: Avon Books, 1993.

Sarno, John E. *Healing Back Pain: The Mind/Body Connection.* New York: Warner Books, 1991.

Sears, Barry. *Mastering the Zone.* New York: Regan Books/HarperCollins, 1997.

Sivananda Yoga Center. *The Sivananda Companion to Yoga.* New York: Simon & Schuster, 1982.

Smedes, Lewis B. *Forgive and Forget: Healing the Hurts We Don't Deserve.* New York: Pocket Books, 1986.

Starlanyl, Devin. *The Fibromyalgia Advocate: Getting the Support You Need to Cope with Fibromyalgia and Myofascial Pain Syndrome.* Oakland, CA: New Harbinger, 1998.

Starlanyl, Devin, and Mary Ellen Copeland. *Fibromyalgia and Chronic Myofascial Pain Syndrome: A Survival Manual.* Oakland, CA: New Harbinger, 1996.

Swami Satchidananda. *Integral Yoga Hatha.* New York: Henry Holt, 1970.

Thomas, Clayton L., ed. *Taber's Cyclopedic Medical Dictionary,* 14th edition. Philadelphia, PA: F. A. Davis, 1981.

Wagner, James K. *Blessed to Be a Blessing.* Nashville, TN: Upper Room Publications, 1991.

Weil, Andrew. *Natural Health, Natural Medicine.* Boston, MA: Houghton Mifflin, 1990.

Weschler, Toni. *Taking Charge of Your Fertility: The Definitive Guide to Natural Birth Control and Pregnancy Achievement.* New York: HarperCollins, 1995.

Wilson, E. Denis, M.D. *Wilson's Syndrome: The Miracle of Feeling Well.* Orlando, FL: Cornerstone Publishing, 1996. (Ordering information: [800] 621-7006)

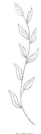

Notes on Contributors

Eduardo Barrera's exercise program, Muscle Balance and Function Development, which was originally developed in San Diego, California, by Geoff Gluckman, allowed him to return to function after he himself developed FM. In addition to teaching this beneficial program of exercise and stretching at the GravityWerks clinic in Seattle, Washington, he lectures at support groups and professional organizations across the United States. Eduardo can be reached at GravityWerks, 3272 California Ave., Seattle WA 98116, (206) 933-1411.

Dr. Kim Bennett has been a physical therapist since 1980. She was trained as an anatomist before her love of anatomy took her into physical therapy. Her practice emphasizes the care of multisystem orthopedic problems. She has specialized in treating FM for the last eight years and works with arthritis patients as well. She also treats acute and chronic spine and peripheral joint dysfunctions. She can be reached at Olympic Physical Therapy, 515 Minor Avenue, Suite A, Seattle WA 98104, (206) 447-1570.

Dr. Paul B. Brown is a rheumatologist in private practice in Seattle. He serves as attending physician at numerous local hospitals in the Seattle area. He cohosted a talk show, "Health Talk," on Washington State public television from 1993 to 1995 and currently serves as an expert witness at trials in support of people with FM. He can be reached at Arnold Medical Pavilion, 1221 Madison Street, Suite 918, Seattle WA 98104, (206) 587-0693.

Dr. Dedra Buchwald is director of the University of Washington Chronic Fatigue Clinic at Harborview Medical Center in Seattle. She is also the director of the CFS Cooperative Research Center at Harborview. She is currently conducting research on CFS and related disorders. These studies, which receive funding from the National Institutes of Health, focus on the prognosis of CFS; CFS and FM in twins; possible links between CFS, mononucleosis, and the Epstein-Barr virus; and cognitive behavior therapy, as well as virological factors. She has also been involved in research on the effects of FM on sleep, as well as the development of a registry for physicians with CFS and FM. She can be reached at Box 359780, 325 9th Avenue, Seattle WA 98104, (206) 731-3111.

Rich Carson founded Pro Health, Inc., a patient-owned nutritional supplement company. Pro Health also publishes *Healthwatch* [see Resources], which has a distribution of more than 200,000. Profits from the sale of the supplements are donated to CFS research. Rich can be contacted at Healthwatch, 1187 Coast Village Road #1-280, Santa Barbara CA 93108-2794, (800) 366-6056, Fax (805) 965-0042.

Vijay Elarth is a certified yoga instructor. He smoked cigarettes for twenty-five years before he began yoga, but quit smoking immediately after his first class and hasn't smoked since. He is the owner of and can be reached at Karuna Integral Yoga Center, 2118 NE 61st Street, Seattle WA 98115, (206) 527-0975.

Noreen Flack is a licensed massage practitioner who works at Seattle Acupuncture Associates, which treats many FM and CFS patients. Many of her patients have had success with acupuncture, massage, and other complementary therapies. She can be reached at Seattle Acupuncture Associates, 515 Minor Avenue, Suite 16, Seattle WA 98104, (206) 622-0246.

Dr. Robert Freitas is a chiropractor and owner of Sea View Chiropractic Clinic in West Seattle. He attended Western States Chiropractic College in Portland, Oregon. (Receiving a chiropractic degree in that state requires eight years of college, including a bachelor's degree in chemistry or one of the sciences plus four years of chiropractic college. A board examination, the National Board of Basic Sciences, similar to the one that dentists and medical doctors take, is required to graduate.) He can be reached at Sea View Chiropractic, 5617 California Avenue SW, Seattle WA 98136, (206) 938-3175.

Kim Ivy practiced martial arts for twenty years and became involved with *tai chi* and *chi kung* after she was injured in a serious car accident. Acupuncture, massage therapy, *tai chi*, and *chi kung* helped restore full mobility in her body. Kim first started teaching *tai chi* and *chi kung* about ten years ago. She has also taught in a retirement community, working with arthritic residents. She can be reached at Embrace the Moon, 5340 Ballard Ave. NW, Seattle WA 98107, (206) 789-0993.

Joleen Kelleher has been involved primarily in caring for people who have cancer; for thirteen years she served as director of nursing at Fred Hutchinson Cancer Research Center in Seattle. For the past eight years she has studied complementary therapy, homeopathy, herbal therapy, nutrition, yoga, and the powerful effects of people taking responsibility for their health and learning that their bodies are designed for health. Joleen believes in finding natural ways to support the process of healing. You can reach her through The Light Institute for Health, P.O. Box 526, Olga WA 98279, (360) 376-6821.

Carol Landis, D.N.Sc. is a professor at the University of Washington who studies sleep dysfunction in patients with FM. She completed her graduate training at the University of California at San Francisco School of Nursing and her postdoctoral training in sleep research at the University of Chicago. She can be reached at BNHS, Box 357226, University of Washington, Seattle WA 98195, (206) 616-1908.

Dr. Cathy Lindsay runs a busy osteopathy practice and lives in Seattle. She is a graduate of the College of Osteopathic Medicine of the Pacific in Pomona, California. She can be contacted at 914 East Miller Street, Seattle WA 98102, (206) 325-5430.

Dr. Kate Lorig is an associate professor at Stanford University and lectures throughout the country on strategies for managing chronic illness. She is coauthor of *Living a Healthy Life with Chronic Conditions* and the *Arthritis Help Book*. She is a consultant to the Arthritis Foundation on implementing curricula to teach arthritis self-management throughout the world. She can be reached through Stanford University School of Medicine, 1000 Welch Road, Suite 204, Palo Alto CA 94304, (650) 723-7935.

Joanna McKee and **Stich Miller** are cofounders of a medical marijuana distribution business, Green Cross, and they vow to continue to supply medical marijuana to sick patients in spite of federal law. They can be contacted at Green Cross, P.O. Box 47347, Seattle WA 98146, (206) 762-0630.

Dr. Philip Mease is a well-respected rheumatologist in private practice in Seattle. He is also a clinical associate at the University of Washington and is the director of clinical research at Minor & James Medical. He can be reached at 515 Minor Avenue, Suite 300, Seattle WA 98104, (206) 386-9500, or through his Web site at http://weber.u.washington.edu/~pmease

Cornelia Duryeé Moore has been a practicing Christian for twenty-three years. She is currently studying to be an Episcopal priest and has counseled

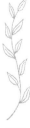

people in matters of spirituality and healing prayer for the last fifteen years. She practices healing prayer in her own life and has seen it work in the lives of others. You can write to her at corneliamoore@hotmail.com.

Cherste Nilde is a craniosacral practitioner in Hawaii. She can be reached at 45-535 Luluku Road #B73, Kaneohe HI 96744.

Maureen Sweeny Romain is a psychotherapist who has worked with people who are post-transplant and have developed chronic illnesses. Over the last three years, she helped establish a wellness center, the Light Institute for Health, which focuses on adjunct therapies (such as nutrition, yoga, homeopathy, and psychotherapy) for people who are experiencing catastrophic or chronic illnesses. She can be reached at 2512 Williams, Bellingham WA 98225, (360) 734-3314.

Morris Rosenberg has served as King County Superior Court Family Law Commissioner ProTempore. He is a member of the Trial Lawyers Association, the Washington State Trial Lawyers Association, and the American Bar Association Section on Dispute Resolution. He serves on the Executive Committee of the King County Bar Association, ADR Section, and he has been special district counsel for the Washington State Bar Association since 1984. He can be reached at Mussehl and Rosenberg, 1111 Third Avenue, Suite 2626, Seattle WA 98101, (206) 622-3000.

Dr. Devin Starlanyl, besides coauthoring *Fibromyalgia and Chronic Myofascial Pain Syndrome: A Survival Manual* and authoring *The Fibromyalgia Advocate: Getting the Support You Need to Cope with Fibromyalgia and Myofascial Pain Syndrome*, has produced a video, *Myofascial Pain Syndrome: A Guide to the Trigger Points*. Although she is not currently in private practice, she has a more than full-time job answering questions, researching, and writing articles on the subject. She lives in New Hampshire and has a Web site at http://www.sover.net/~devstar

Dr. Dennis Turk has been involved in numerous aspects of pain research for twenty-five years. He is a fellow and diplomat of the American Board of Psychotherapists, a founding member of the American Pain Society, a charter member of the International Association for the Study of Pain, and a fellow of the Academy of Behavioral Medicine Research. He received his Ph.D. from the University of Waterloo in Ontario, Canada. He can be

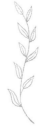

reached through the Department of Anesthesiology, University of Washington, Box 356540, Seattle WA 98195, (206) 616-2626.

Don Uslan cofounded the Center for Comprehensive Care with Dr. Philip Mease. The clinic offers physical and occupational therapy as well as acupuncture, massage, and herbal medicine. Mental-health services are available, including social work, psychology, biofeedback, stress management, and pain management. All work is coordinated among the treatment providers. The clinic also provides vocational rehabilitation for people with FM. He is a certified rehabilitation counselor with the Commission on Rehabilitation Counselor Certification and the rehabilitation consultant to the Chronic Fatigue Clinic at the University of Washington. He can be reached at Northwest Counseling Associates, 515 Minor Avenue, Suite 18, Seattle WA 98104, (206) 628-3400.

Sara Wicklein, a licensed acupuncturist, is in private practice in Seattle. She graduated from acupuncture school at Bastyr University in 1993. She can be reached at 444 NE Ravenna Boulevard #106, Seattle WA 98115, (206) 525-3030.

Dr. Rebecca Wynsome is a licensed primary-care physician in Seattle whose practice focuses on the health-care needs of women. She has discussed her treatment methods on radio programs and ABC's *Good Morning America*. She is a graduate of Bastyr University and a member of the American Association of Naturopathic Physicians. She was a consulting advisor to the author of *Taking Charge of Your Fertility*. Dr. Wynsome is currently working on a new book, *Correcting Imbalanced Hormones*. She can be reached at 150 Nickerson Street, Suite 211, Seattle WA 98109, (206) 283-1383.

Dr. Michael Young lives in Tacoma, Washington. He is author of the book *Unbelievable Pain*, due in bookstores in December 1999, and can be reached at VA Puget Sound Health Care System, American Lake Division, 9900 Veteran's Drive SW, Tacoma WA 98493, (253) 582-8440.

Index

A

acetaminophen, 253

aching muscles, 30, 37

acid reflux, 121

Acupuncture Association of Washington, 239

acupuncture, xii, 19, 65, 66, 67, 68–71, 166, 242

addiction, narcotic, 183–184

adenosine triphosphate (ATP), 202

Adrenal Stress Index, 134

aerobic conditioning, xii, 19, 242

alcohol abuse, 32

Alexander Technique, 142, 242

allergies, food, 122, 123

Alpha Stim, 240

alternative therapies, 5

Ambien, 95, 182, 253

American Association for Chronic Fatigue Syndrome, 239

amitriptyline, 18, 253

analgesics, narcotic, xii, 18, 46, 180–200, 253, 254

anemia, 31

anesthetics, 253, 254

anorexia nervosa, 32

antianxiety drugs, 50

antidepressants, xi, 18, 46, 49, 78, 182, 186, 205, 253, 254

antidyskinetic, 254

anti-inflammatory drugs, 33, 46, 186, 253

antioxidants, 47

antispasmodic drugs, 253

antiviral drugs, 33

anxiety, as root of fibromyalgia and chronic fatigue syndrome, 77–78

Arnica montana, 72

Arthritis Foundation, xiv, 154, 239, 240

arthritis, 124, 242; degenerative, 17, 19; rheumatoid, 17, 19

Ashii points, 70

aspirin, 253

astragalus, 67

attorney, hiring, 219–220, 224–227

autoimmune disorders, 96, 243

B

B vitamins, 168

baclofen, 253

Bentyl, 19, 253

biofeedback, xii, 19, 243

bipolar disorders, 32

bladder, irritable, 10, 17, 246

blue-green algae, 47

bowel, irritable, 10, 17, 122, 246

breath, shortness of, 37

breathing, deep, 26, 161

bulimia, 32
bupropion, 254
BuSpar, 50, 253
buspirone, 253

C

calcium citrate, 50
cancer, 33
candida, 123, 243
car accidents, 10–11
carbidopa-levodopa, 254
carbohydrates, 27, 121
carisoprodol, 254
Center for Fatigue Sciences, 239
CFIDS & FM Health Resource, 216, 240
CFIDS Association of America, 239
CFIDS Chronicle, 238
Chemical Injury Information Network, 239
chemical sensitivity, 41, 247
chest pain, 37
chi kung, 65, 67–68, 74–76, 204, 243
chi, 65–66, 243
chiari malformation, 215
Chinese herbs, 47
Chinese medicine, 65–76, 243
chiropractic care, xii
chiropractic therapy, xii, 26, 48, 243; finding a doctor, 54; techniques, 55–59
chlamydia pneumoniae, 200

Chlorazopate, 50
chocolate therapy, 166
cholac lactulose syrup, 47
chondoitin, 124
Christian healing, 97–103
chronic fatigue syndrome, causes of, 10–11, 33–34; definition, xi, 1, 244; diagnosis of, 9–17, 30–34; symptoms of, 10, 30, 32, 37–44; treatment of, xx; conventional therapies, 45–51
cleansing, spiritual, 166
clonazepam, xi, 253
clorazepate dipotassium, 254
co-enzymes, 202
cognitive behavioral modification techniques, xii, 33, 244
cognitive difficulties, 10, 37
colonic cleansings, 166
concentration, difficulty, 37
constipation, 17, 37, 121
coping mechanisms, 82–83, 88, 201
CoQ10, 50
Correctol, 47
cortisol, 134
cortisone injections, 46
craniosacral manipulation, 60, 170–173
cyclobenzaprine, 253
cystitis, 17
Cytomel, 253

D

dairy products, 125

Deltasone, 253

dementia, 32

depression, xi, 30, 31, 32, 33, 37; as root of fibromyalgia and chronic fatigue syndrome, 77–78

dermatomyocytis, 96, 244

Desyrel, 253

detoxification, 121

DHEA, 50, 134, 135, 186

diarrhea, 17, 37

diclofenac, 254

Dicyclomine, 49, 253

diet, 27; high fiber, 19; protein, 28–29

disability benefits, 112–116, 217–223

discrimination, 4

disorientation, 38

dong quai, 67

Doxepin, 18, 254

drug abuse, 32

Duragesic, 46, 188, 253

E

Edwards, Blake, 213

Effexor, 186

eggplant, 124

Elavil, 48, 186, 253

elimination diet, 245

emotional trauma, 10–11

Endocet, 253

endocrine conditions, 18

Endodan, 253

environmental illness, 41, 247

epileptic seizures, 28

Epstein-Barr virus, 31

Estratest, 124

evening primrose oil, 47

exercise, 33, 88, 139–164, 204

F

Family Leave Act, 112

fasting, 126–128

fatigue, 10, 17, 30, 37; diagnostic criteria, 31

Feldenkrais method, 204, 245

fentanyl transdermal, 253

fever, low-grade, 37

fiber, dietary, 125

Fibromyalgia Health Letter, 238

Fibromyalgia Network, 138

Fibromyalgia Times, 238

fibromyalgia, causes of, 10–11; definition, xi, 1, 245; diagnosis of, 9–36; symptoms of, 10, xx, 37–44; treatment of, 17–20, 26–27; conventional therapies, 45–51; occurrence of, xi, 1

Fibroplex, 135

filtering, 38

flaxseed oil, 125

Flexeril, 18, 46, 95, 186

flu symptoms, 30

fluoxetine, 254

folic acid, 27

foods, problem, 124–125

formaldehyde, 41

G

gabapentin, xii, 253
gardening, 89
gastrointestinal problems, 37
general assistance, 221
ginger root, 67
gingko biloba, 47, 124
glucosamine, 124
Green Cross, 190, 192–196
growth hormone, 209, 211; defi-
    ciency, xii
guaifenesin, 26, 47, 253

H

Hashimoto's disease, 245
headaches, 10, 30, 37
healing, Christian, 97–103
healing, natural, 119–138
healing, spiritual, 166
Health Points, 238
Healthwatch, 238
heart palpitations, 37
heat, 48
herbs, Chinese, 66–67
herpes virus, 31
HHV6 (human herpes virus six),
    214–215
homeopathy, 72–73, 246
hormone balancing, 133
hot-tub therapy, 166
housing, subsidized, 113
hyaluronic acid, 25
hydrocodone, 254
Hypericium perfoliatum, 73

hyperthyroidism, 246
hypnosis, xii
hypothyrodism, 246

I

ibuprofen, 18, 253
ice packs, 48
Imitrex, 253
immune system, 33
INFA News, 238
infections, 31
insurance benefits, 48, 113, 223
intimate relationships, 81
irritable bladder syndrome, 10, 17,
    246
irritable bowel syndrome, 10, 17,
    122, 246

K

Kaopectate, 47
Ketorolac, 254
Klonopin, 253

L

lactose intolerance, 126
laughter, 88
legal rights, 217–231
LEM, 212–213
levothyroxine sodium, 254
Levsinex, 19, 253
licorice, 67

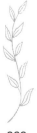

Lidocaine, 19, 253
linden flowers, 67
Lioresal, 253
liothyronine sodium, 253
low natural killer cell syndrome
    (see chronic fatigue syndrome)
lupus, 17
Lyme disease, 18, 93–94, 246–247
lymph glands, 31; tender, 10
lysocyamine, 253

M

macrobiotic diet, 122
magnesium, 27, 47, 50, 186
magnet therapy, 166
malic acid, 41, 47, 50
marijuana, medical, 182–183,
    184–185, 190–194
Marinol, 185
massage therapy, 19, 26, 166, 169,
    176–179, 247
Medicaid, 113
Medicare, 113
meditation, 19, 166
melatonin, 68
memory, poor, 10
Metagenics, 241
methadone, xii, 46, 181, 182, 189,
    253
methocarbamol, 254
methotrexate, 254
microcurrent treatments, 168–167
migraine headaches, 48

migraine medications, 253
mindfulness, 92
Minnesota Multi-Phasic Personality
    Inventory, 2
morphine, 253
Motrin, 253
Movement Therapy, 144–149
moxa, 66
MS-Contin, 46, 253
MSM (methyl sulfonyl methane),
    47
multiple sclerosis, 33
Muscle Balance and Function
    Development, 141, 144–149,
    247; exercises, 147–148
muscle pain, 37
muscle relaxants, 18, 19, 46, 253,
    254
music, 89
myalgic encephalomyelitis, 33
myofascia, 23
myofascial pain, 23–27
myofascial release therapy, 19, 247

N

NADH, 202
Naprosyn, 46, 253
naproxen, 18, 253
narcotic analgesics, xii, 18, 46,
    180–200, 253, 254
narcotic patch, 189, 253
National CFIDS Foundation, 239

National Fibromyalgia Research Association, 239
natural healing, 119–138
naturopathy, 123, 133–136, 247
nausea, 121
nefazodone, 254
neuralgia, 248
neurocirculatory asthenia, 33
Neurontin, 4, 46, 253
neurotransmitters, 11, 25, 258; disorders, 200
Norflex, 46, 254
nortriptyline, 18, 254
nutrition, 65, 120–130, 167, 248

O

obesity, 32,
opiates, 183–187, 248, 253, 254
Optimum Health Institute of San Diego, 240
orphenadrine citrate, 254
orthotics, 166; mouth, 169
osteopathy, 52–64, 248–249; techniques, 59–61, 166
Oxycodone, 46, 181, 185, 188, 253
Oxycontin, 4, 46, 197, 254
oxygen therapy, 167

P

pain management, 2, 46
paint thinner, 41
Pamelor, 254

paroxetine, 254
Paxil, 18, 254
peanuts, 125
peppers, 124
Percocet, 187, 254
Percodan, 254
perfumes, 41
pesticides, 41
petrochemicals, 41
phosphoric acid, 25
physical therapy, xii, 48, 139, 150–155, 249
pineal gland, 68
podiatry, 249
poetry, 82
potatoes, 124
prayer, 84
prayer, healing, 98–103
prednisone, 253
Proactive Living Program, 117
Procaine, 19, 254; injections, 46
Pro-Energy, 47
prolactin, 201, 209, 211
protein, 122
Prozac, 18, 43, 46, 254
prunes, 125
psychological aspects, fibromyalgia and chronic fatigue syndrome, 205–208
psychotherapy, 48, 90–93, 249

Q

questionnaire, 7–8
quinolinic acid, 25

R

reflexology, 166
relationships, 80–81
relaxation, 19; progressive, 152
research, chronic fatigue syndrome,
    212–216
restless-leg syndrome, 61
rheumatology, 249
Rheumatrex dp, 254
Rhus toxicodendron, 73
Robaxin, 18, 186, 254
Roxicet, 254
Roxicodone, 254
Roxiprin, 254

S

schizophrenia, 32
sciatica, 249–240
sedatives, 253
self-management techniques, 202,
    203–205
self-talk, 204
serotonin, 250
serotonin reuptake inhibitors, 33,
    186
sertraline, 254
Serzone, 18, 46, 182, 254
Sinemet, 46, 254
Sinequan, 254
Skelaxin, 186
sleep apnea, xii, 20, 250
sleep disorders, 10, 16, 18, 25, 30,
    37, 209–211; research, 209–211

sleeping aids, xi, 253
sleeping positions, 24
smoke, 41
smoking, 27
Social Security Administration, 240
Social Security Disability
    Advocates, 240
Social Security disability benefits,
    113, 217–223
Soma, 18, 186, 254
Somato-Emotional Release, 171
sore throat, 10, 30, 37
spiritual counseling, 97–103
spirituality, 77–105
steroids, 19, 46
stress eating, 121
stress, 18, 33, 81, 152
stretching, 19, 26
subluxations, 56
Substance P, 11, 200, 250
sumatriptan, 38, 253
support groups, 83, 84, 240
support systems, 20
surgery, 48
swimming, 19
Synthroid, 254

T

Tae-Bo, 142
tai chi, 19, 65, 68, 74–76, 142, 204
temporomandibular joint disorder
    (TMJ), 21, 251
tender points, xi, 9, 10, 251; injec-
    tions, 19, 251

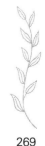

tenderness, 17
tennis balls, 166
therapies, conventional, 45–51
thyroid conditions, xii, 15,18, 31, 245, 251, 253, 254
tomatoes, 124
Toradol, 46, 254
toxicity, 25
tramadol, 254
Tranzene, 254
trauma, physical, 10–11
Trazodone, 18, 46, 48, 186, 253
tricyclics, 33
trigger points, myofascial, 23–24, 56, 251
turmeric, 67
Tylenol, 186, 254

U

UltraClear Sustain, 121
Ultram, 46, 49, 50, 186, 187, 254
urination, frequent, 37

V

Vicodin, 46, 254
visualization, 166, 204
vitamin B complex, 47
vitamin B1, 27
vitamin B12, 27
vitamin B6, 27
vitamin C, 47
vitamin deficiency, 27

vitamin E, 47
vocational rehabilitation, 115–119, 251
Voltaren, 254
volunteering, 89

W

walking, 19
Washington Intractable/Chronic Pain Advocacy, 240
water aerobics, 166
Wellbutrin, 18, 46, 254
Wilson's Syndrome Foundation, 240, 252
Wisconsin Viral Research Group, 239
women and chronic fatigue syndrome, 30, 82; and fibromyalgia, 1, 82, 211
work, 106–119
workplace modification, 112

Y

yoga, 142, 159–162, 252

Z

Zantac, 41
zinc, 47
Zoloft, 18, 46, 50, 254
zolpiden, 253

RUNNING ON EMPTY: The Complete Guide to Chronic Fatigue Syndrome (CFIDS) 3rd edition. *by* Katrina Berne, Ph.D.

Although it can be difficult to diagnose, CFIDS is a real, biologically-based disease with options for effective treatment and management. Written by an expert who has CFIDS herself, this book offers clarity, hope, and support. It includes summaries of recent medical findings on treatments, ideas on living with the disease, and intimate stories of other sufferers. The accurate information and sympathetic, upbeat tone make this an invaluable book for CFIDS patients and a complete reference for the health care professionals who treat them.

"Well-researched, well-organized, and eminently readable, this book should prove quite a boon to CFIDS sufferers." — Booklist

336 pages ... 3rd Edition ... Paperback $14.95 ... Hard cover $24.95

GET FIT WHILE YOU SIT: Easy Workouts from Your Chair *by* Charlene Torkelson

Here is a total body workout that can be done right from your chair, anywhere. It is perfect for office workers, travelers, and those with age-related movement limitations or special conditions. The book offers three programs. *The One-Hour Chair Program* is a full-body, low-impact workout that includes light aerobics and exercises to be done with or without weights. *The 5-Day Short Program* features five compact workouts for those short on time. Finally, *the Ten-Minute Miracles* is a group of easy-to-do exercises perfect for anyone on the go.

160 pages ... 212 b/w photos ... Paperback $12.95 ... Hard Cover $22.95

WOMEN LIVING WITH MULTIPLE SCLEROSIS *by* Judith Lynn Nichols and Her Online Group of MS Sisters

Judith Nichols was first diagnosed with MS in 1976 and cofounded an online support group of women who helped each other cope with the day-to-day challenges of MS. In this book, members of the group share intimate, emotional accounts of their experiences with MS. Some stories are painful, some are funny, often they are both. The range of deeply personal concerns includes family reactions to a diagnosis of MS, workplace issues and relationships, sexuality and spirituality, depression and physical pain, loss of bladder and bowel control, and assistive devices and helpful tools. All topics are discussed freely and frankly, in the way closest friends do.

288 pages ... Paperback ... $13.95

ORDER FORM

10% DISCOUNT on orders of $50 or more —
20% DISCOUNT on orders of $150 or more —
30% DISCOUNT on orders of $500 or more —
On cost of books for fully prepaid orders

NAME

ADDRESS

CITY/STATE   ZIP/POSTCODE

PHONE   COUNTRY (outside of U.S.)

TITLE	QTY	PRICE	TOTAL
Alternative Treatments...(paperback)		@ $15.95	
Alternative Treatments...(hard cover)		@ $25.95	

Prices subject to change without notice

Please list other titles below:

		@ $	
		@ $	
		@ $	
		@ $	
		@ $	
		@ $	
		@ $	

Check here to receive our book catalog ☐   FREE

Shipping Costs:
First book: $3.00 by book post ($4.50 by UPS, Priority Mail, or to ship outside the U.S.)
Each additional book: $1.00
For rush orders and bulk shipments call us at (800) 266-5592

TOTAL	_____
Less discount @_____%	(_____)
TOTAL COST OF BOOKS	_____
Calif. residents add sales tax	_____
Shipping & handling	_____
TOTAL ENCLOSED	_____

Please pay in U.S. funds only

☐ Check ☐ Money Order ☐ Visa ☐ Mastercard ☐ Discover

Card #_____ Exp. date_____

Signature_____

Complete and mail to:
Hunter House Inc., Publishers
PO Box 2914, Alameda CA 94501-0914
Orders: (800) 266-5592   email: ordering@hunterhouse.com
Phone (510) 865-5282 Fax (510) 865-4295
☐ Check here to receive our book catalog

ATF 10/99